The American Medical Women's Association

Guide to Cancer and Pain Management

Medical Co-editors
Roselyn Payne Epps, M.D., M.P.H., M.A., F.A.A.P.
Susan Cobb Stewart, M.D., F.A.C.P.

A Dell Book

Published by
Dell Publishing
a division of
Bantam Doubleday Dell Publishing Group, Inc.
1540 Broadway
New York, New York 10036

This material was originally published along with other material in THE WOMEN'S COMPLETE HEALTHBOOK published by Delacorte Press.

Illustrations by Wendy Frost

ISBN: 0-440-22250-8

Reprinted by arrangement with Delacorte Press

Printed in the United States of America

Published simultaneously in Canada

November 1996

10 9 8 7 6 5 4 3 2 1

OPM

KNOWLEDGE MEANS EMPOWERMENT. TEST YOURSELF.

1. Working out with weights can help sagging breasts. True or false?
2. Is most breast cancer genetically linked in families?
3. Is breast cancer the leading cause of death from cancer? Is it the most common cancer in women?
4. Can you get information about cancer faxed to you?
5. Is some pain "all in your head" or purely psychological?
6. Is surgery, such as cutting a nerve, an effective treatment for pain?
7. What is the common over-the-counter drug that will affect men and women differently?

ISN'T IT IMPORTANT THAT YOU HAVE THE FACTS? YOUR LIFE AND YOUR HEALTH MAY DEPEND ON THEM.

Answers:

1. *False. No kind of exercise can help.*
2. *No. 80% is not.*
3. *No, lung cancer is. However, it is the most common cancer in women.*
4. *Call 301-402-5874 from a touch-tone phone and follow the directions.*
5. *A very small percentage—5 percent. Most pain is real.*
6. *No, it is only used as a last resort.*
7. *Acetaminophen (Tylenol).*

Other books by the American Medical Women's Association

THE WOMEN'S COMPLETE HEALTHBOOK
THE AMWA GUIDE TO NUTRITION AND WELLNESS
THE AMWA GUIDE TO PREGNANCY AND CHILDBIRTH
THE AMWA GUIDE TO FERTILITY AND REPRODUCTIVE HEALTH
THE AMWA GUIDE TO EMOTIONAL HEALTH
THE AMWA GUIDE TO SEXUALITY

COMING SOON

THE AMWA GUIDE TO AGING
THE AMWA GUIDE TO EARS, NOSE AND THROAT
THE AMWA GUIDE TO CARDIOVASCULAR HEALTH
THE AMWA GUIDE TO INTERNAL DISORDERS

The AMWA Guide to Cancer and Pain Management

Roselyn Payne Epps, M.D., M.P.H., M.A.,
and Susan Cobb Stewart, M.D.

Persistent pain often triggers suspicion of cancer. While cancer is only one of the many potential causes of pain, both pain management and cancer awareness are issues of central importance to women. Women need a definitive resource for accurate, dependable, and up-to-date information. *The AMWA Guide to Cancer and Pain Management* tells you what you need to know about the process of detecting cancer and various methods of dealing with pain, as researched by the American Medical Women's Association (AMWA), the most historic and prestigious association of women physicians in the United States.

The AMWA believes that women must avoid a disease-oriented approach to health and focus on maintaining optimal health on a daily and long-term basis. The more one knows about one's body and its functions, the better equipped one will be to safeguard good health by eating properly and exercising regularly. The content of *The AMWA Guide to Cancer and Pain Management* is organized into four major sections, each of which stresses the importance of preventive medicine and encourages total body awareness to manage health problems.

Part I, Cancer in Women, alerts the reader to the warning signs of cancer and the factors that place a woman at risk for developing the disease, covering every aspect from genetics and environmental hazards to lifestyle and diet. Being familiar with the symptoms of cancer can prompt women to seek medical attention and potentially speed up the process of early professional diagnosis. Although each woman's case requires individual treatment, a general discussion of the various available methods such as radiation, surgery, and chemotherapy will make women aware of their options.

Part II, The Breast, outlines the structure and function of the breast. The highly specialized cells in women's breasts make this area susceptible to the formation of cancerous growths, a fact that helps to explain why breast cancer is the most common form of cancer in women. This section also explores other diseases and conditions that affect breast tissue, such as benign tumors, lactational mastitis, and cysts. The procedures for conducting monthly self-exams are detailed in this chapter.

Part III, Pain Evaluation and Management, describes the mechanism of pain and relates it specifically to the concerns of women. This section includes tips on how to accurately assess and describe pain symptoms when consulting with a physician, which will greatly speed up the process of diagnosing illness and disease. It can also contribute to the effectiveness of deciding how to administer relief, whether it's traditional medicine that employs surgery and medication, or alternative medicine that uses natural healing approaches such as massage, relaxation therapy, and acupressure. This section covers a wide range of different pain management techniques—from psychological counseling to prescription narcotics—to help women decide which approach is best for them.

Part IV, Managing Medication, describes the ways that women are affected by various medications. There are many factors that influence the effects of drugs: gender, age, food, and lifestyle (including alcohol, caffeine, and nicotine intake), weight, menstrual cycles and pregnancy, other prescriptions being taken, and so on. Women need to be aware of how drugs will help or harm them as they attempt to manage pain using prescriptions or over-the-counter medications. This section includes charts demonstrating a wide range of drug interactions, as well as important consumer information regarding proper storage and handling, and how to decode the cryptic abbreviations—such as *t.i.d.* ("three times daily") or *p.c.* ("after meals")—listed on the labels of medication bottles.

The AMWA Guide to Cancer and Pain Management provides authoritative information that all women need to cope with the difficult issues of cancer, terminal illness, and pain. It illuminates the health concerns unique to women of the 1990s and offers sound medical advice. Supported by the expertise and experience of the American Medical Women's Association, *The AMWA Guide to Cancer and Pain Management* is a sensitive and comprehensive approach to health maintenance and wellness for women of all ages.

CONTENTS

PART IV
MANAGING MEDICATION
Jean A. Hamilton, M.D., and
Kimberly A. Yonkers, M.D.

The American Medical Women's Association

Guide to Cancer and Pain Management

PART I

Cancer in Women

Claudia R. Baquet, M.D., M.P.H.

Cancer is characterized by an uncontrolled growth and spread of abnormal cells in the body. If not caught early, this proliferation of abnormal cells—called a tumor—can result in death. You should be aware, however, that cancer is not a hopeless disease, but one that can be cured with prompt treatment. Recent advances in cancer therapy have led to nearly 50% of cancer patients remaining alive and free of disease some 5 years after the initial diagnosis.

Cancer occurs in larger numbers among the elderly. It is much more common in people over 65; about 73 million Americans are eventually expected to develop cancer in their later lives. Lung cancer is the leading cause of cancer-related deaths in both men and women, followed by breast cancer in women. The incidence rates and the death rates vary in men and women and in different ethnic groups, based on the type of cancer.

CAUSES OF CANCER

Why does cancer occur? What triggers an occurrence? The reasons are still largely unknown, although the mechanisms of the disease have long been recognized.

The body renews and replaces its cells through a constant process of cell division and growth. Cells exist, repair themselves, die, and are reborn. Old tissues are replaced with new, injuries are repaired, and the body grows and develops. Normally, the body has control mechanisms that limit abnormal cell growth. Cancer cells, however, continue to grow without restraint, dividing many more times than do normal cells. The abnormal cells form tumors, which compete with normal, healthy tissue for nutrients.

Tumors can be benign (harmless) or malignant. Benign tumors can be removed with surgery and usually do not recur. Malignant tumors, on the other hand, can grow, invade, and destroy nearby areas of the body. They can spread, or metastasize, to distant organs and form new tumors. If malignant tumors aren't removed or killed early in their development, they can spread to other parts of the body.

Some cancers spread quickly, whereas others develop slowly. Because cancers can be most successfully treated before they spread (metastasize), it is important to be aware of cancer warning signs and steps that can be taken for early detection of the disease.

METHODS OF EARLY DETECTION

The American Cancer Society has identified certain warning signs that should alert you to see your doctor promptly (see "The Seven Warning Signs of Cancer"). None of these signs necessarily means that you have cancer, but each one is important and warrants immediate medical attention. Pain is seldom a symptom of early types of cancer, so don't wait until it hurts if the other symptoms don't disappear on their own.

Certain tests can also help detect cancer in early stages. These screening tests are often done routinely for people who may have symptoms of a disease and for those who have risk factors, such as age and family history. Every woman should have a physical examination annually and undergo the following routine screening tests as needed.

- Pelvic exam and Pap test (annually after age 18 or once sexual activity has begun) to detect cancer of the cervix, ovary, or uterus.
- Mammography (every 1–2 years until age 40–49; yearly thereafter) to detect cancer of the breast. High-risk women may benefit from earlier screening.
- Fecal occult blood test (annually after age 50) to detect hidden blood in the stool, which may be a sign of cancer of the colon and rectum.
- Sigmoidoscopy (every 3 to 5 years after age 50) to detect changes in the colon or rectum that could be a sign of colon and rectal cancer.

These tests may be done earlier in women who have special risks. For instance, if you have a family history of cancer of the breast or colon, you will benefit from having tests to detect these diseases more than women who have no family history of disease. Colonoscopy, a test used to view the inside of the entire colon, is recommended in women age 40 and older who have had inflammatory bowel disease or who have a family member who had cancer of the colon or rectum at an early age.

Be alert to any changes in your body. Besides scheduling a yearly pelvic exam, you should regularly examine your breasts. Many breast lumps have been found through self-examination. It is best to do the breast examination at the same point in your menstrual cycle each month (or on the same day of the month if you're postmenopausal), because breast tissue changes with your cycle. It will be easier for

THE SEVEN WARNING SIGNS OF CANCER

1. Change in bowel or bladder habits
2. A sore that does not heal
3. Unusual bleeding or discharge
4. Thickening or lump in the breast or elsewhere
5. Indigestion or difficulty swallowing
6. Obvious change in a wart or mole
7. Nagging cough or hoarseness

you to detect anything unusual if you follow this suggestion. Check out other areas of your body, including your skin, for any suspicious signs.

Have your mouth checked periodically by a dentist. In addition, use a mirror to examine your mouth. Changes in the color of the gums, lips, or cheeks as well as sores, swelling, bleeding, or thickening of any tissue should be reviewed by your doctor.

RISK FACTORS OF CANCER

About 80 percent of all cancers may be related to the things we eat, drink, and smoke and to the quality of our environment and workplace. Repeated and long-term contact with cancer-causing agents (carcinogens) can damage cells or change cells that are already damaged and lead to cancer. For example, tobacco smoke is one of the most potent carcinogens, and it acts with other elements, such as alcohol, to increase the risk of certain cancers.

Tobacco

Smoking is a major risk factor for cancer. The risk of dying from lung cancer is 12 times greater in a smoker than in a nonsmoker. Overall, smoking causes 30 percent of all deaths from cancer. In addition to contributing to lung cancer, it also increases the risk of cancers of the cervix, mouth, throat, esophagus, pancreas, bladder, and possibly the stomach. Smokers also have a higher rate of cardiovascular and respiratory disease. Household members of smokers are also at risk for cancer.

If you smoke, quit. As soon as you stop smoking, your risk of cancer decreases.

Diet

A high-fat diet has been linked to certain types of cancer, including cancer of the breast, colon, rectum, and ovaries. Obesity has been linked to increased cancer death rates. The exact link between diet and cancer is not clear, but most health practitioners agree that it is best to eat a variety of foods, to limit saturated fats and cholesterol, and to eat foods high in fiber. Eating fresh fruits and vegetables daily may decrease your risk of cancer by as much as 50 percent. An increased daily intake of vitamins A, C, and E may also boost your protection against lung cancer.

Sunlight

One of the most common forms of cancer in the United States is skin cancer, which is caused by exposure to ultraviolet (UV) radiation from the sun.

Repeated exposure to the sun may be especially harmful for people who have fair skin or who burn or freckle easily. Take steps now to avoid the sun, especially between the hours of 10:00 A.M. and 2:00 P.M., when the sun's rays are strongest. If you are out during those times, wear protective clothing, including a hat. Use sunscreen to block the UV light. Remember, a tan is really the body's attempt to protect itself against the sun.

Alcohol

Cancers of the mouth, throat, esophagus, and liver occur more often among heavy drinkers, especially those who smoke as well. Alcohol also poses a number of other health problems. If you regularly drink more than two drinks a day, you should probably consider cutting back or stopping drinking altogether.

Chemicals

Exposure to certain industrial agents or chemicals increases the risk of various types of cancer. Exposure to these chemicals may occur in the workplace, outdoors, or at home. They include:

- Asbestos fibers
- Nickel, chromate, and vinyl chloride
- Solvent cleaners, cleaning fluids, and paint thinners
- Lawn and garden chemicals (pesticides and fungicides)

Avoid inhaling any of these chemicals, especially in areas that are not well ventilated. Read labels carefully and avoid having these agents come in contact with your skin or household items.

Hormones

Certain cancers are stimulated by an excess of the female hormone estrogen. Estrogen occurs naturally in reproductive-age women. It is also the main component of birth control pills and hormone-replacement therapy after menopause. Birth control pills have not been linked to cancer in most women, however, and they may even protect against some types of cancer. Replacement of estrogen alone can increase the risk of endometrial cancer in postmenopausal women, but when it is combined with the hormone progesterone, the risk is lowered. Before taking estrogen, discuss the risks with your physician.

Genetics

Some cancers may be inherited. The risk of breast, colon, and skin cancer, for instance, is higher in some families than in others. Your risk for these cancers is high if you have a first-degree relative (mother, father, sister or brother) who developed one of these cancers. If you have close relatives who have had cancer, tell your doctor. He or she may advise that you receive regular checkups and tests.

TYPES OF CANCER

Cancer in women can be nongynecologic or gynecologic. *Nongynecologic* cancers occur in both men and women. *Gynecologic* cancers, however, are unique to women; they occur in the female reproductive and genital organs. (Although breast cancer can occur in both men and women, it is considered here as a gynecologic cancer, because it is much more common in women than in men.) For more details about all of these cancers, see the chapters where the specific body parts are discussed. (See Fig. 1.1)

Nongynecologic Cancers

Lung

Today, lung cancer is the most common cause of cancer death in American women, resulting in the death of 59,000 women in 1994. The rate of occurrence as well as the death rate from lung cancer is on the rise in both white and African-American women.

The main cause of lung cancer is cigarette smoking. Other less common causes are exposure to radon gas, asbestos, and radiation.

The specific warning signs of lung cancer are as follows:

- A cough that won't go away
- Sputum streaked with blood
- Chest pain
- Repeated attacks of pneumonia or bronchitis

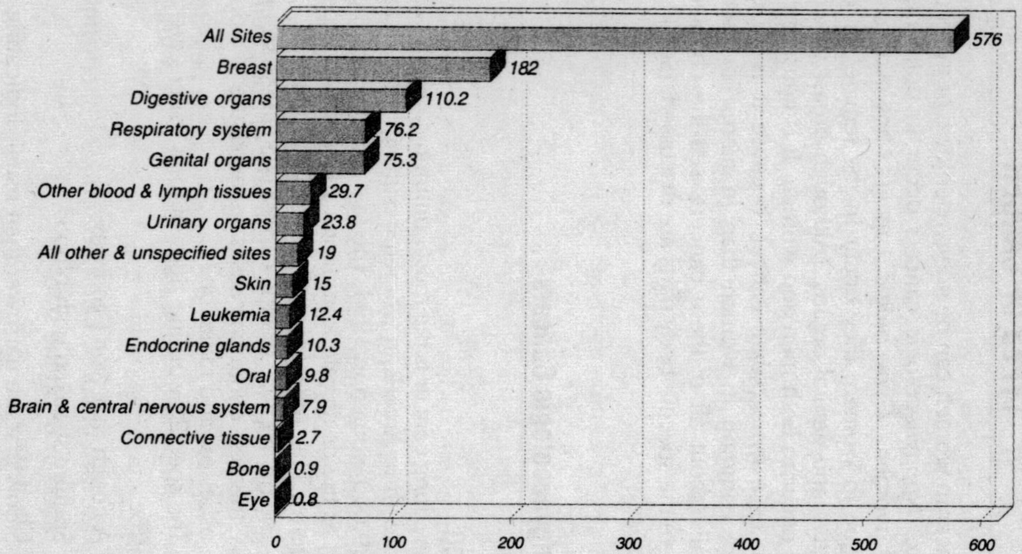

Figure 1.1 Estimated New Cancer Cases and Deaths in Women, 1994.

There are no screening tests for lung cancer, and it can be difficult to diagnose. Nearly 90 percent of patients diagnosed with lung cancer receive care too late to be cured. Diagnosis is based on chest X rays, examination of the cells in the sputum, biopsy of the suspicious area, and imaging tests of the bronchial tubes. Survival rates are low and based on the stage of disease. Surgery is the main form of treatment, followed by chemotherapy. Some cancers will be treated by radiation therapy. The best way to combat lung cancer is prevention by stopping smoking.

Colon and Rectum

Cancer of the colon (the large bowel) and rectum (the last 8 to 10 inches of the large bowel, which leads to the anus) is the second most common cancer in women. Although the death rate from colon and rectum cancer is decreasing in white women, it is remaining steady for African-American women. This form of cancer occurs more often in older women, in those who have a history of inflammatory bowel disease, and in women who have a family history of cancer of the colon or rectum. A diet high in saturated fat and low in fiber appears to increase the risk of this disease, and increased daily intake of fiber, fruits, and vegetables seems to protect against it.

Cancer of the colon and rectum can be detected early. The following persistent symptoms are warning signs of a possible problem:

- Diarrhea or constipation (recurring or alternating)
- Blood in or on the stool
- Stools that are narrower than usual, indicating obstruction

- General abdominal discomfort (bloating, fullness, or cramps)
- Frequent gas pains
- A feeling that the bowel doesn't empty completely

These symptoms could be a sign of a number of things, so it's important to ascertain the cause without delay. The diagnosis is based on a physical examination and tests that detect blood in the stool or growths in the colon or rectum. Sometimes a piece of a growth can be removed for further study (biopsy). The most common treatment for bowel cancer includes surgical removal of the diseased area, and follow-up chemotherapy may be recommended.

Bladder

Each year, more than 13,000 American women will be diagnosed with bladder cancer. If the disease is treated early, the cure rate is good. Cancer of the bladder is twice as likely to occur in women who smoke as in women who don't smoke. The main symptom is blood in the urine and the need to urinate more often than normal. Pain rarely occurs in the early stages, and there may be no symptoms at all.

Diagnosis is based on physical examination, laboratory tests, and imaging studies. A urine sample may reveal cancer cells. Since the cancer usually occurs inside the bladder, a test may be done using a thin lighted tube that is inserted inside the bladder. A sample of any growth may be removed for further study. Bladder cancer is usually treated surgically.

Skin

Skin cancer is the most common form of cancer in the United States, with about 700,000 new cases annually. It is estimated that 40 to 50 percent of Americans who live to age 65 will have skin cancer at least once. Caused by exposure to ultraviolet light, skin cancer occurs more often in regions that traditionally have more sunlight. Basal cell carcinoma, a slow-growing cancer that usually does not spread to other parts of the body, accounts for more than 90 percent of all skin cancers. It usually appears as pale bumps or red scaly patches. Squamous cell skin cancer can spread to other areas and must be removed surgically. Multiple melanoma is invasive and life threatening. It first appears as a molelike growth that gets bigger, darker, and more inflamed. (See Fig. 1.2)

Warning signs of skin cancer include:

- A change in the size or color of a mole or wart
- Scaliness, oozing, or bleeding
- Itchiness, tenderness, or pain in a bump or a mole
- A sore that does not heal

Regular self-examination is the best way to detect skin cancers. Inspect all moles carefully and look for any changes. Examine all parts of the body, because melanoma can appear in places that have not been exposed to sunlight. The cure rate is nearly 100 percent if skin cancers are treated before they spread.

Pancreas

The pancreas, a large gland located behind the stomach and in front of the spine, makes enzymes that digest food as well as insulin, which controls the amount of sugar in the blood.

Cancer of the pancreas is a common cause of death in women. It is known as a *silent* disease, because there are no symptoms in the early stages. As

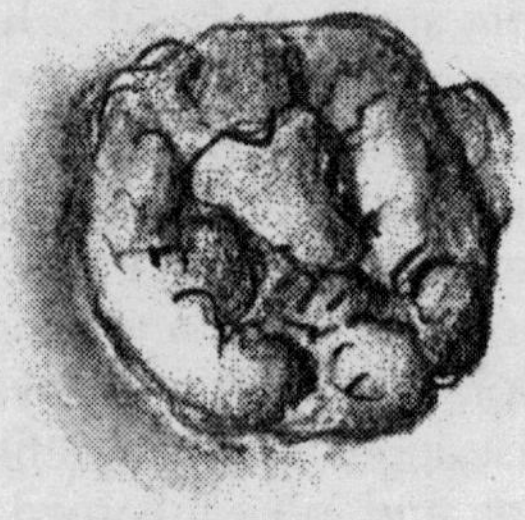

Figure 1.2 Skin Cancer.
Basal cell cancer is the most common type of cancer and looks like pale bumps or red patches.

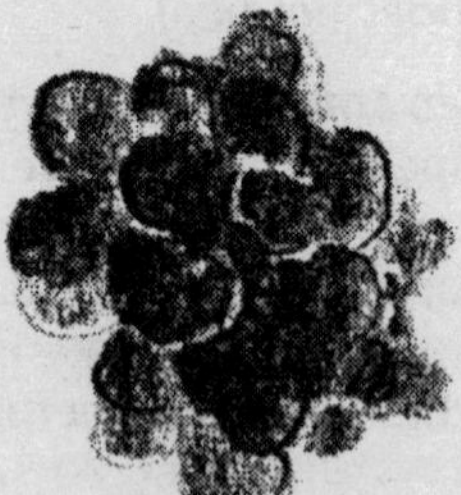

Melanoma is a less common but more severe type of skin cancer that looks like a mole but grows bigger and darker.

a result, the cancer has often spread by the time it is diagnosed, which makes for low survival rates. Symptoms are pain in the upper abdomen and sometimes the back, nausea, loss of appetite, weight loss, and weakness.

Oral

Cancers of the mouth, lips, gums, cheeks, teeth, jaw, and tongue are usually found in people over age 45. The best way to detect oral cancer is through self-examination. Look for the following warning signs:

- A sore that bleeds easily and doesn't heal
- A lump or thickening
- A red or white patch that doesn't go away
- Difficulty chewing, swallowing, or moving tongue or jaws

Women who smoke, especially if they also drink alcohol, are at an increased risk for oral cancer.

Diagnosis is established by taking a biopsy of any lump or abnormal area and examining it under a microscope. Imaging tests also may be done to see if the disease has spread to other parts of the body. If caught early, many of these cancers can be cured.

Gynecologic Cancers

Breast

Breast cancer is occurring in epidemic proportions in the United States. About one of every nine women will develop breast cancer during her lifetime. African-American women, who are less likely than white women to develop breast cancer, are more likely than white women to die from it. Formerly, it had been thought that African-American women postponed seeing a doctor or did not have access to care, resulting in the disease being diagnosed in later stages. Recent research, however, indicates that a more aggressive form of the disease may afflict African-American women, particularly younger ones.

Women who have a mother or a sister who has had breast cancer are at increased risk of getting the disease. The risk is also higher in women who have not had children or who had children later in life. Breast cancer has also been linked with alcohol use and a high-fat diet.

The best way to detect breast cancer is by doing a monthly self-examination, seeing a doctor annually for an examination, and by having periodic mammograms. The warning signs of breast cancer are

- Changes in the breast that don't disappear—a lump, thickening, swelling, or dimpling
- Irritation of breast skin
- Nipple distortion, retraction, or scaliness
- Discharge from the nipple

The earlier breast cancer can be found and treated, the better the chance of cure. Breast cancer can spread to the bones, liver, lungs, or brain, making it very difficult to treat in later stages.

The first stage in diagnosis is feeling for any breast lumps. Your doctor may use a needle to withdraw fluid or a piece of the lump so that it can be studied in a laboratory. Treatment of breast cancer depends on how advanced the cancer is at the time of diagnosis.

Cervix

The cervix, the narrow neck of a woman's uterus, can go through a series of changes that eventually can lead to cancer. Cervical cancer is the third most common form of cancer of the female genital tract and accounts for 19 percent of these cancers. Cervical cancer occurs almost twice as often in younger African-American than in age-matched white women; over the age of 65, African-American women develop cervical cancer about three times more often than white women. Death rates follow similar patterns, with African-American women dying more often from the disease.

Risk factors for cancer of the cervix include having sex at an early age, having multiple sexual partners, and smoking. Women without any of these risk factors can also develop cervical cancer, however.

A precancerous or localized condition of the cervix can develop over time into invasive cancer. There may be no warning signs with early cervical cancer. More advanced cervical cancer can be signaled by abnormal bleeding or vaginal discharge. Changes in the cervix can be detected through regular Pap tests. Precancerous changes in the cervix can be treated before they become cancerous.

To confirm the diagnosis, a biopsy is done. A sample of tissue from the cervix is removed and studied under a microscope. If detected early, the cancer can be removed surgically. For prevention, always have a Pap smear test done at least once a year after the age of 18.

Endometrium (Uterus)

Cancer of the uterus accounts for 5 percent of all cancers in women and is the most common gynecological cancer. Most cancers of the uterus occur in the endometrium, the lining of the uterus.

Endometrial cancer occurs most often in older women; it is rare before age 40. Cancer of the endometrium is more likely to affect women who are infertile, began menstruating at an early age, don't have children, have menstrual problems, and go through menopause at a later age. Other risk factors include obesity, diabetes mellitus, hypertension, and use of estrogen. Gallbladder disease and thyroid disease may also be associated with increased risk.

The most common symptom of cancer of the endometrium is abnormal bleeding or discharge from the vagina. Because this disease often occurs in women around the age of menopause, they may mistake this symptom for a menstrual period. Any bleeding or discharge that appears after menopause should be checked by a doctor.

Cancer of the endometrium is diagnosed by removing a piece of the lining of the uterus for further study. A hysterectomy (removal of the uterus) is the usual treatment.

Ovary

The ovaries are located on either side of the uterus; each month during ovulation one of the ovaries releases an egg. These glands also produce estrogen. Cancer of the ovary is the second most common gynecologic cancer and the fourth-leading cause of death from cancer among women.

Risk factors for cancer of the ovary include a family history of the disease. It generally develops after menopause and is seen more often in women who have had no children or who had trouble conceiving. It is often hard to detect until it is in the advanced stages, when the following warning signs occur.

- Discomfort in the pelvic region
- Indigestion, gas, or bloating
- Pain during intercourse
- Abnormal vaginal bleeding
- Pain and swelling in the abdomen

There is no good method of screening for cancer of the ovary, although the use of two tests, ultrasound and a blood test for a protein called CA125, show promise. Any abnormality should be checked by a doctor. Imaging tests may be done to get a better idea of the size of a growth. Surgery to remove the ovary, and any other affected organs, is an important part of treatment.

Vulva and Vagina

Cancer of the vulva and vagina are rare and occur most often in older women. Warning signs include a lump or sore on the vulva (external genitals) or in the vagina.

Risk of vaginal cancer is increased after radiation of the cervix, chronic irritation, and uterine exposure to the hormone DES. Diagnosis is determined by removing a sample of tissue for further study. If detected in the early stages, cancers of the vulva and the vagina can be treated successfully.

TYPES OF CANCER TREATMENT

Although a diagnosis of cancer is serious, it no longer carries the dire consequences it once did. Nearly 50% of all patients diagnosed with cancer can now be cured because of advances in early detection and treatment. The type of treatment is based on the stage of disease. It can involve surgery, radiation therapy, chemotherapy, or a combination of these. Emotional support is invaluable in helping patients with cancer deal with the physical and psychological aspects of their disease.

At the time of diagnosis, the extent of the disease is determined. Called *staging,* this is a useful way to determine whether cancer is localized or has spread to other areas. Additional staging is used to determine types of treatment and possible outcomes. One method of classification is *historical stage,* which relates the extent of cancer at the time of diagnosis to the natural history of the disease. The *localized stage* refers to a cancer that is confined to its place of origin. The *regional stage* refers to disease that has spread beyond its place of origin to surrounding areas. The *distant stage* is cancer that has spread extensively to distant tissues or organs.

For localized cancer, surgery is often used to remove the affected tissues. During the surgery, a lymph node or nodes may be removed for examination to see if cancer has spread to the lymphatic system, where it can be spread to other parts of the body.

Radiation therapy is another form of local therapy. Treatment can be directed to particular areas of the body, or radioactive units can be implanted at the site of the cancer. For other cancers, the whole body

THE AFTERMATH OF CANCER: WHAT YOU CAN DO

Cancer changes the life of the person who has it as well as the lives of the family and friends of that person. If you suffer from cancer, you may have initially reacted to the disease with anger and denial and now feel a range of emotions from hope to despair. More important, you may feel that you have suffered physical and emotional losses that you find hard to deal with and that prevent you from moving ahead to continue on with your life.

Support groups, psychologists and psychiatrists, and families and friends are important recovery resources.

may receive radiotherapy. Radiation can be used occasionally before surgery to shrink tumors or after surgery to destroy any remaining cancer cells.

Drug therapy, known as chemotherapy, uses drugs to destroy cancer cells. These chemicals interfere with the cells' ability to grow and multiply. The drugs may be administered orally or intravenously. Chemotherapy can destroy healthy cells as well as cancer cells. Side effects of chemotherapy vary and are strongly related to the specific drug or drugs given as well as the type and extent of disease.

Antihormonals block the body's production of specific hormones. The growth of some cancers is stimulated by hormones, and antihormonal drugs limit that stimulation. One such drug is tamoxifen, which is used to treat some breast cancer. Because this drug interferes with the actions of estrogen, women who take it may develop symptoms of menopause.

Some types of cancer therapy have side effects, some more severe than others. Many side effects are temporary, and many can be successfully managed so that the patient is as comfortable as possible.

THE FUTURE OF CANCER RESEARCH AND CANCER CARE

Research in new areas of cancer prevention and treatment is ongoing. One area of research is directed toward examining cancer at the molecular level. By identifying genes that may cause cancer or may make one more susceptible to cancer, scientists hope to be able to target people who are at risk so they can receive early treatment and may even be able to avoid getting cancer at all.

Other research efforts are being directed toward antioxidants, chemicals that consume free radicals, which are waste products produced by our bodies. Some evidence suggests that free radicals may cause cell damage and degeneration. Other research is trying to find ways to boost the body's natural immune response, so it can fight cancer wherever it appears in the body.

PART II

The Breast

Janet Rose Osuch, M.D., F.A.C.S.

Breasts are an anatomic feature unique to a woman and her role as a mother. They are able to respond to stimulation—cold, sex, or a nursing baby. Because of the breasts' ability to be stimulated during sexual activity and because of the importance society has placed on them, the breasts are intimately tied to femininity.

The breasts serve a very important function—the feeding of a baby. Breast milk is the best food for a newborn. It's often been imitated but never equaled.

Of the various conditions that can affect the breasts, the most feared is breast cancer, the most common cancer in women. However, a woman has a number of ways to detect breast cancer early, when it can be treated with the most success.

This chapter describes the structure and function of the breasts, some common conditions that may occur, and the diagnosis and treatment of breast conditions. It also describes ways a woman can help keep her breasts healthy.

STRUCTURE AND FUNCTION OF BREASTS

The breast rests on the *pectoral* (chest) muscle. The interior of the breast is made up of fat, *stroma* (connective tissue), *lobules* (glands that produce milk), *ducts* (the tubes to carry milk to the nipples), and blood vessels (see Fig. 2.1 A and B).The only muscles in the breast are the tiny ones near the nipple. You can see them at work when the nipple becomes erect from stimulation or cold; the purpose of this function is to make the nipple more prominent so a baby can nurse. The darkened area around the nipple is called

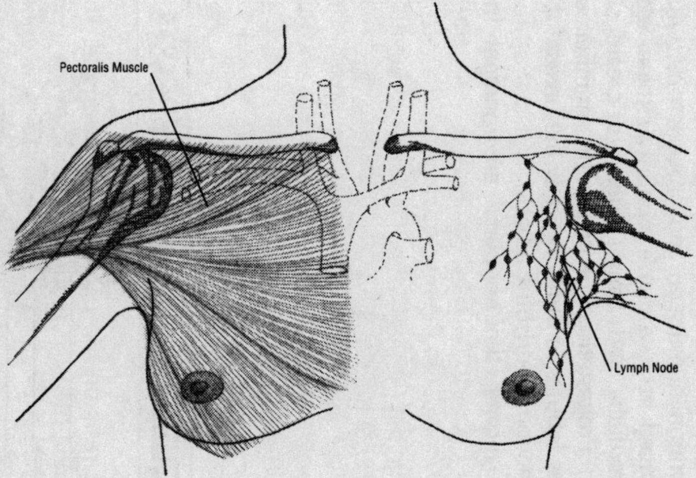

Figure 2.1A. The Breast
The breast is located on top of the pectoralis muscle of the chest (left). The tissue around the breast and under the arm contains clusters of lymph nodes, which are infection-fighting organs in the lymphatic system (right).

the *areola*; it may be pink, brown, or black, depending on the woman's coloring. The areola contains small glands that lubricate the nipple during breastfeeding. Sometimes, quite normally, these appear as raised bumps on the areola.

Breast development and function depend on two major hormones, estrogen and progesterone, which are produced in a woman's ovaries. Estrogen elongates the ducts and causes them to create side branches. Progesterone increases the number and size of the lobules in order to ready the breast for its major function, nourishing a baby.

Each month, the hormonal environment in a

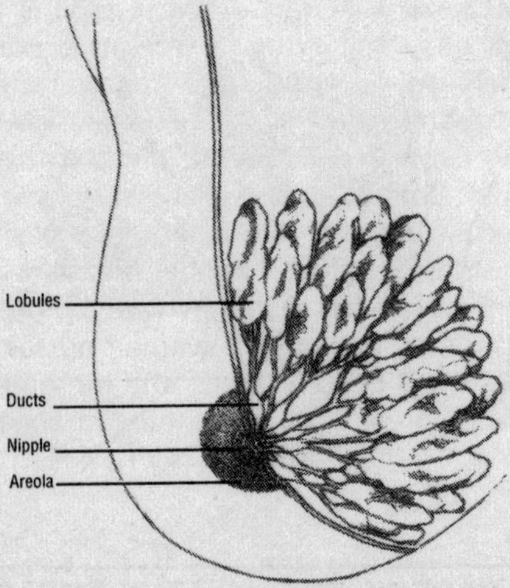

Figure 2.1B. Anatomy of the Breast
The breast is made up of lobules that are connected to ducts that lead to the nipple in the center of the areola.

woman's body changes according to the phase of her menstrual cycle. Between the first day of a woman's menstrual period and about 14 days later, when an egg is released from her ovary (ovulation), the breasts are in a relatively dormant state. After ovulation, which occurs midcycle, progesterone makes the breast cells grow and the blood vessels enlarge and fill with blood. At this time, the breasts often become engorged with fluid and may be tender and swollen. This is especially true the week before menstruation.

LACTATION

The biological function of the breast is to feed a woman's offspring. When a woman becomes pregnant, her breasts grow larger and firmer as milk begins to form (see Fig. 2.2). This growth continues until the baby is delivered. If a woman nurses her baby, her breasts will remain firm and become engorged with milk throughout the day. When a woman stops breast-feeding, her breasts will sag and may become smaller than they were before pregnancy. Regardless of whether a woman nurses her baby, her breasts will become softer and more droopy as a result of the pregnancy. All of these changes are normal.

CARE OF THE HEALTHY BREAST

A woman's day-to-day routine can include specific ways of supporting her breasts. Many women wear a

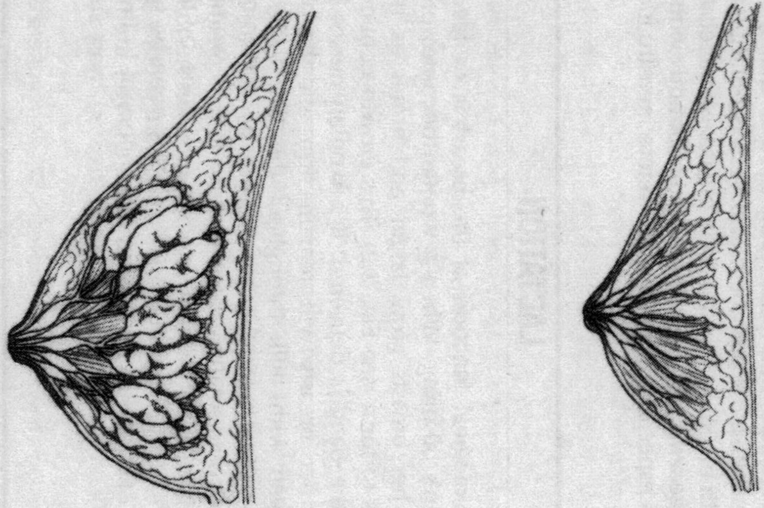

Figure 2.2. Effects of Pregnancy
During pregnancy (left), breasts become larger, and milk glands increase to prepare for breast-feeding.

bra for support and comfort. If a woman exercises, she may want to wear a special sports bra for comfort, to keep her breasts from moving around during exercise. There is no exercise, however, that will keep breasts from sagging, because this is a normal part of aging. Exercising can tone the chest muscles under the breasts, but there is no muscle in the breast itself to be toned, to grow, or to stop sagging. Exercising can help reduce overall body weight, and this in turn may reduce the size of breasts; in turn, weight gain often results in breast enlargement.

Some women use lotions on their breasts, but there is no need to treat breast skin differently from the skin of the rest of the body. Women who expose their breasts to the sun should always wear sunscreen. The skin of the breasts is just as vulnerable to cancer as the skin on any other part of the body.

Cancer Screening

The single most important way to promote breast health is with regular breast cancer screening. Screening is looking for signs of disease in women with no symptoms. Some screening is done by the woman herself, and other screening is done by her health care professional. Both are important in finding cancer early, when it can be treated most successfully.

Compared with other cancers, breast cancers are quite slow growing in most women. On average it takes between eight and ten years for one breast cancer cell to grow and multiply to the point where it can be detected as an abnormal mammogram (8 years) or a lump in the breast (10 years).

BREAST SCREENING GUIDELINES

Guidelines for breast screening depend on a woman's age. Recommendations for how often screening should be done are shown in the chart below. Clinical examination is an exam by a physician or nurse.

Age	Self-Examination	Clinical Examination	Mammography
20–39	Monthly	At least every three years	Not recommended
40–49	Monthly	Annually	Every year or every other year
50 and up	Monthly	Annually	Annually

Breast cancer screening involves self-examination, clinical breast examination (physical examination of the breast by a physician or nurse), and mammography (breast X rays). Recommendations about the type and timing of screening by health care providers are hotly debated in the medical community, centering primarily on when routine mammography should begin and how often it should be done in women of specific ages. AMWA recommends the schedule shown in the chart. These are the guidelines promulgated by the American Cancer Society. A woman and her doctor should decide together how often she should be screened.

One important consideration is a woman's fami-

RISK FACTORS FOR BREAST CANCER

Increased Risk

- Family history of breast cancer, especially in mother, daughter, or sister
- Older age (the older the woman, the higher the risk)
- No pregnancies or pregnancy after age 30
- Menstrual periods starting at a young age (under 10)
- Late menopause (over 52)

ly history. A woman with a first-degree relative (a mother, sister, or daughter) with breast cancer is at greater risk of developing breast cancer herself. She will need to be screened earlier and more often. Other factors that affect a woman's risk for cancer are shown in the box on risk factors. But 80 percent of women who develop breast cancer have no family history, so it is vital that all women undergo regular breast cancer screening. With early detection, breast cancer can be curable. Breast cancer screening could save your life.

Breast Self-Examination

If you don't already examine your breasts monthly, start now. If you examine yourself every month at the same time of the month, you can become familiar with what your normal breast tissue feels like. If you are still menstruating, choose the week after your period for your self-exam. If you no longer menstruate, choose any time of the month (the first Saturday, for example, or your birth date) and follow that schedule. You may also want to examine your breasts soon after your health care provider does, since everything should be normal then.

Breast self-examination is simple to do. The basic steps are shown in the box on page 33. Your doctor or nurse also can show you how.

At first, self-examination can be confusing. What should you expect to feel? The normal breast of a woman who has not gone through menopause feels bumpy. This is because the milk producing cells form little "nests" between the fat cells. These nests increase in size at ovulation, which is why breasts are more bumpy at that time in the cycle. Following menopause, the nests of cells shrink and just the fat is left behind. That's why normal breasts in postmenopausal women feel smoother.

One way to tell what's normal and what's not is to compare the two breasts side by side. For example, if you feel something "different" in the tissue near the underarm, examine the same spot by the opposite breast. If the areas feel the same, there is usually little need for worry. If the other side doesn't feel the same, however, there may be cause for concern. Call your doctor with any doubts or concerns.

Clinical Breast Examination

A clinical breast examination can be done by a woman's regular doctor or by a nurse in the doctor's office. The exam is most often done along with a routine pelvic exam and Pap test (the test for cervical cancer). If your doctor doesn't routinely examine your breasts, you should insist that she or he do so; if this isn't possible, find a different doctor.

BREAST SELF-EXAMINATION

1. Stand or sit in front of a mirror with your arms at your sides. Look for any changes in the breast, such as dimpling, redness, or different breast size or shape (A).
2. Look for the same signs with your hands on your hips (B) and then with your arms over your head (C).
3. Lying on your back, put your right arm over your head and use your left arm to examine your right breast. Palpate (press with the fingers), using dime-sized circles, moving in ever smaller circles from the outside of the breast toward the nipple. Cover the entire breast (D).
4. Feel the underarm area.
5. Switch to the other side and do steps 3–4 on that side. (See Fig. 2.3, A–D)

The clinical breast exam is much like the breast self-exam you should do each month. It can vary a bit from doctor to doctor, however. A woman should try to schedule her breast exam for the week after her period, especially if she is worried about the results of her self-exam. This way, her breasts are less likely to be tender or swollen, and any abnormalities will be easier to notice.

Mammography

The third line of defense in maintaining breast health is mammography, or breast X ray. It can be used for routine screening in women without symptoms or, if a problem is suspected, to aid in diagnosis. In mam-

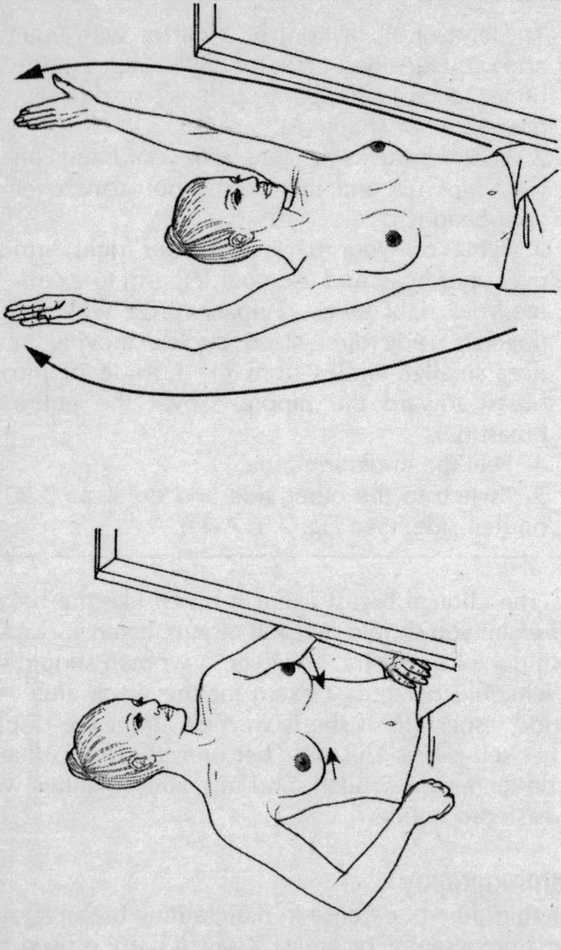

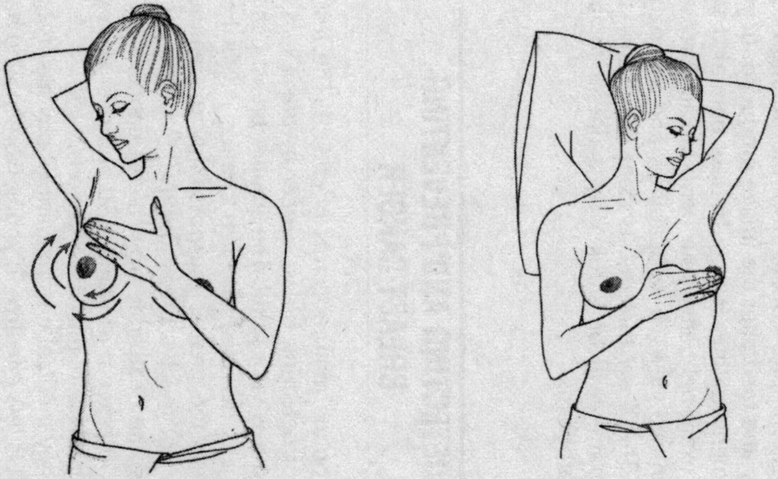

Figure 2.3. Breast Self-Examination
Breast self-examination should be performed monthly. In order to detect changes, a woman should become familiar with the normal shape and feel of her breasts. (See the box on page 33—"Breast Self-Examination.")

mography, the breasts are placed, one at a time, between two plastic plates. Pressure is applied to make the breast as thin as possible. Some women find this pressure painful, but it's necessary. The more the breast is compressed, the lower the radiation dose necessary and the better the image produced. (If you are still menstruating, it may be less painful if you have the exam right after your period.) Each breast is X-rayed in two views, a vertical view and a horizontal view. The X ray that results from the exam—the mammogram—will be studied by a doctor for any signs of problems.

DETECTING AND PREVENTING BREAST CANCER

Having routine mammograms is critical. The test is capable of detecting breast cancer before it can be felt, when it is very small. The smaller breast cancer is when it is detected, the less chance it will have spread, and the greater the possibility of treatment that does not involve breast removal. Mammograms save lives; the death rate from breast cancer can be reduced 30 percent in women 50 and over who get mammograms at regular time periods.

Like any medical test, mammography has its limitations. It is less effective in young women who have what radiologists (physicians who specialize in use of X rays) refer to as dense breasts. The breasts are normal, but they do not photograph well on the X ray. When milk-producing cells and ducts are X-rayed, they appear white—the same color as an abnormality such as cancer cells. Therefore, the denser the woman's breasts, the less likely it is that a breast cancer will be detected by a mammogram. There is at least a 15 percent false-negative rate with mammography. This means the mammogram appears to show no abnormality when in fact there is a problem. In these cases, breast cancer will be diagnosed by physical examination alone.

Generally, mammogram results are classified into one of the following groups:

- Normal (no abnormalities on the X ray)
- Benign abnormality (changes seen, but they are likely not cancer)
- Indeterminate (changes seen are probably benign but possibly cancerous)
- Suspicious
- Cancer until proven otherwise

Depending on your results, there are a number of tests that may be done to diagnose the problem. You and your doctor will decide together what steps to take.

For a mammogram to be most accurate, it's critical that the X-ray equipment be of the best quality. Federal legislation in 1992 set laws on equipment quality. To find out about mammography machines in your area, call the American Cancer Society at 1–800–ACS–2345. The society can give you the names of mammography facilities in your area that are accredited by the American College of Radiology.

The need for breast cancer screening never stops. The chances of developing breast cancer rise as a woman ages. Therefore, it should always be a part of her life, just like Pap tests and trips to the dentist.

Cancer Prevention

While methods for detection are well studied, less is known about breast cancer prevention. Current research could take years to yield answers. One promising area is the use of the drug tamoxifen to prevent breast cancer. This synthetic hormone is also used to treat breast cancer. Researchers are also looking for a link between low-fat diet and lower rates of breast cancer. This is suggested from animal tests, but tests in women are not yet conclusive.

DISEASES AND CONDITIONS OF THE BREAST

Breast Cancer

The single greatest health concern regarding breasts is breast cancer. Here are some facts:

- Depending on how long a woman lives, her lifetime risk of getting breast cancer can be as high as 1 in 8.
- In the 1990s, almost 2 million women will be diagnosed with breast cancer.
- Breast cancer is the most common cancer in women.
- Breast cancer is the second-leading cause of death from cancer, after lung cancer.
- Of women diagnosed with breast cancer, 80 percent have no family history or other risk factor except gender and age.

The good news is that early detection may mean cure. Regular breast exams and mammography, as recommended, can catch cancer early, when treatment is more likely to succeed.

Symptoms and Signs of Breast Cancer

There are a number of warning signs of breast problems, many of which are symptoms that a woman can detect herself (see box on page 43). These symptoms do not necessarily mean cancer is present. They are warnings that further investigation is needed.

Breast Lump

Most commonly a woman herself or her partner finds a lump, a hard area of breast tissue that stands out from the normal surrounding breast tissue when that spot is touched or examined. The lump can be as small as the size of a pea. The term "lump" refers to any firm tissue that is not present in the same location in the opposite breast, even if it feels like a thickening rather than an actual lump. Other than the lump, a woman generally will have no symptoms. In some cases, there may be some tenderness near the lump.

Nipple Discharge

If discharge occurs only on nipple stimulation, it is normal. However, if discharge emerges on its own (staining underthings or bedsheets), a woman should see her doctor. A discharge from only one breast is more likely to be a symptom of cancer than if both breasts are involved.

Skin Redness

Redness is always a cause for concern. It can mean an infection or cancer, especially when a woman is not breast-feeding. It should be checked by a doctor.

Breast Pain

In very rare cases, breast pain may indicate cancer, especially when the pain is at the site of a lump or thickening. (See Fig. 2.4)

Nipple Scaling

If the nipple shows flaking or scaling, this can be a symptom of cancer even if no lump can be felt and the mammogram is normal. (See Fig. 2.5)

Skin Puckering or Dimpling

If there is a growth in the breast, it may pull at the breast skin and cause puckers or dimples to appear.

In addition to these symptoms, abnormal results on a mammogram may be a sign that something is wrong. Mammography can sometimes find a tumor

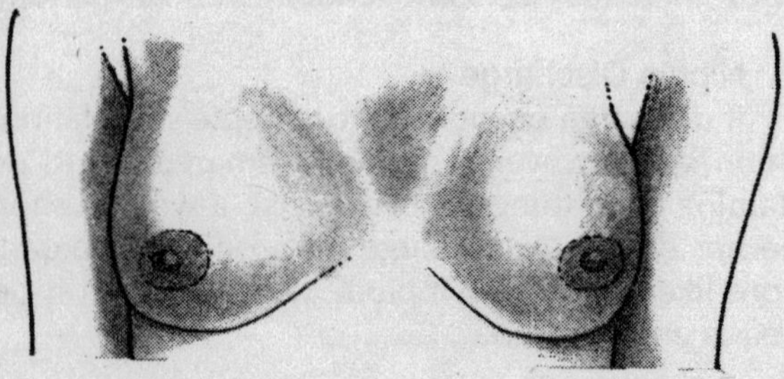

Figure 2.4. Lumps
Breast pain may occur at the site of a lump.

years before the woman herself would feel it. Not every abnormality is cancer; an abnormal mammogram usually suggests that further testing needs to be done. Mammograms will also miss some cancers that can be felt, which is why self-examination and clinical examination by a doctor or nurse are so important.

Diagnostic Procedures

If a woman has any symptoms of cancer or if she has had an abnormal mammogram, a number of procedures may be recommended to diagnose the problem. Some of the more common ones are described here.

Diagnostic Mammography

This procedure uses the same technique as screening mammography. More views of the breast may be needed, so it may take longer. Mammography can also be used to assist with breast biopsy.

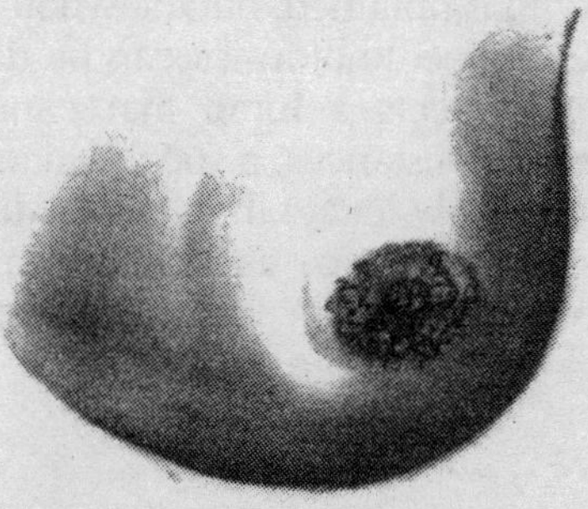

Figure 2.5. Scaling
Scaling of the nipple may be a sign of cancer.

Ultrasound

Ultrasound, a diagnostic test that uses sound waves to make images of tissues, is most commonly done if a mammogram suggests there is a problem. It helps define whether an abnormality is a cyst (fluid-filled sac) or a solid mass.

Fine Needle Aspiration

A small needle is used to withdraw a sample from a breast lump. If the lump is a cyst (fluid-filled sac), aspiration of the fluid will cause the lump to disappear. If the lump is solid, cells can be smeared onto slides for examination in the laboratory. Aspiration does not remove solid lumps, it samples them. The test takes 30 to 60 seconds and can be performed in the doctor's office.

Core Needle Biopsy

This procedure is similar to fine needle aspiration. In it, a larger needle is used because actual breast tissue is removed, not just a few cells. A sample of the lump is obtained, but the whole lump is not removed. Core needle biopsies can be done when a mammogram detects a lump that cannot be felt; under these circumstances, a special machine is necessary to accurately locate the abnormality. This procedure is usually done by a surgeon or a radiologist. The area is numbed with local anesthetic, and the woman will feel some pressure.

Biopsy

In most breast biopsies, the entire lump is removed surgically. The tissue is then studied under a microscope. If a rim of normal breast tissue is taken all the way around a lump (lumpectomy), biopsy can

SYMPTOMS OF BREAST DISEASE

See your doctor if you have any of the following:

- Breast lump
- Nipple discharge that leaves a stain on clothing
- Breast pain
- Skin redness
- Nipple scaling
- Skin puckering or dimpling
- Any unexplained changes in how the breast feels or appears

also serve as part of breast cancer treatment. A breast biopsy is almost always done on an outpatient basis, under a local anesthetic. Some women are given a sedative as well. The procedure takes about an hour.

As a general rule, biopsies are done for these reasons:

- A solid mass persists after a menstrual cycle
- A solid mass is found in a woman who does not ovulate
- Cyst fluid contains blood
- A cyst does not completely disappear after aspiration
- A cyst comes back in the same spot on the breast within two to six weeks of an aspiration
- An asymmetrical abnormality persists

In cases in which breast abnormalities must be removed but cannot be felt on physical examination, a special procedure called a needle localization will be done. During the localization the radiologist finds the abnormality with a needle, takes a mammogram, and repositions the needle as accurately as possible. A wire then replaces the needle, and the patient is sent to the operating room for the biopsy. Sometimes dye is used with the wire or instead of the wire.

Cancer Staging

If the biopsy shows cancer, the pathologist will classify it. Cancer can arise in either of two basic breast parts: the lobules or the ducts.

Once the type of cancer is known, other tests—including lymph node removal in many cases—need to be done to determine if the cancer has spread, and if so, where. (See Fig. 2.6) Tests that may be used include blood tests, chest X rays, and scans of the liver or bone. This process is called staging. It places the cancer in one of 5 groups, ranked 0 through 4. The higher the number, the more the disease has spread and the lower the chance for a cure. Staging helps the doctor decide on the type of treatment that has the best chance for a cure.

Stage 0 is also called cancer in situ. This means that the cancer is still in a strictly limited location. For example, stage 0 cancer of the duct cells is found only in duct cells and is confined to the inside of the duct. In stages 1–4, the cancer is invasive: it has spread outside its place of origin (for example, a cancer that started in the ducts is now in the surrounding tissue).

Most breast cancer (88 percent) is invasive when detected. In stage 1 it is confined to the breast. In

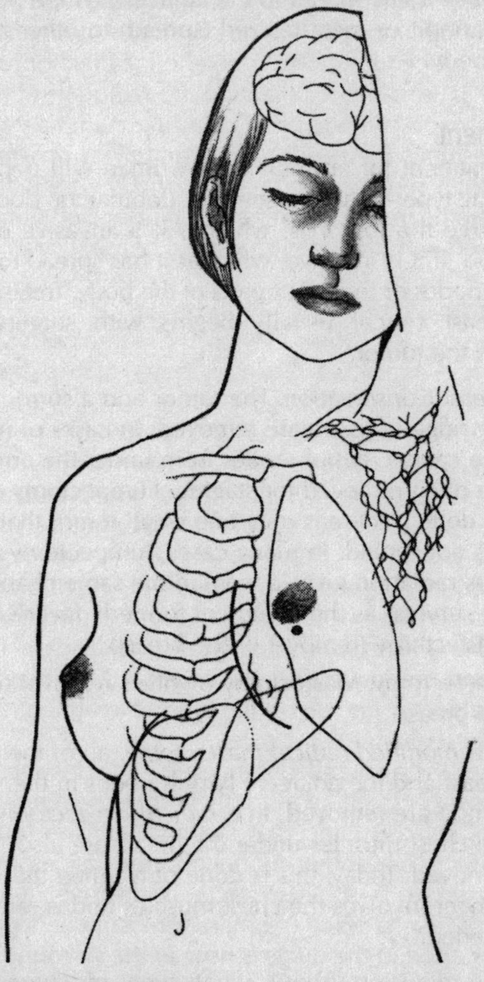

Figure 2.6. Breast Tests
Tests that may be performed in patients with breast cancer include X rays of bone and lungs and liver function tests.

stages 2–4 it has spread to the adjacent lymph nodes in the armpit or metastasized (spread) to other parts of the body.

Treatment

The treatment for an individual woman will depend on what type of tumor she has (lobular or ductal), how large the tumor is, whether it is invasive or in situ, and, if it is invasive, whether it has spread to the lymph nodes or to distant parts of the body. Treatment for breast cancer usually begins with surgery to remove the tumor.

- *Breast Conservation.* The tumor and a surrounding ridge of tissue are removed. In cases of invasive cancer, lymph nodes from under the arm are often removed for staging. Lumpectomy can be done if there is only one small tumor that has not spread. In many cases, lumpectomy plus radiation gives a woman the same chance for survival as the treatment formerly favored, mastectomy (removal of the breast).
- *Mastectomy.* Mastectomy involves removal of the breast.
- In a *modified radical mastectomy,* all of the breast and the adjacent lymph nodes in the armpit are removed. In a *radical mastectomy,* the chest muscles under the breast are also removed. Today, this is done only when the cancer involves the chest muscles and is rarely needed.

The decision about what type of surgery a woman should have can be a difficult one for a woman to make. Once a woman learns that she has cancer, she will usually be able to take time to discuss treatment options with her doctor and her family, and to begin to adjust to the idea of having breast cancer. Today, doctors know that there is no harm in waiting 2 weeks or so to reach a decision the woman prefers. In the past testing and treatment were done together. In this one-step approach, a woman would agree before her biopsy that if cancer were present, the breast would be removed right then, while she was still anesthetized. She had only one surgery, but she also didn't know whether she'd wake up minus a breast.

Following surgery, a woman often will have radiation therapy, especially if she had a lumpectomy. This is done to destroy any remaining cancer cells in the breast. The treatment is begun as soon as the wound from surgery heals. It usually lasts about 6 weeks. Radiation treatment is given by a type of radiologist called a radiation oncologist. Each treatment takes a few minutes. Radiation treatment is local—it is directed to the affected site. Side effects may include a skin reaction such as a sunburn effect or rash, fatigue, and a low white blood cell count (which increases a woman's risk of infection), especially toward the end of treatment. Most women are able to continue their normal routine.

A woman may also have chemotherapy or hormonal therapy, depending on the type of cancer and how far it has advanced. The purpose of these therapies is to treat any possible tumor cells that may have traveled from the tumor site, perhaps to other body parts. These treatments are systemic—they are circulated through the body in the bloodstream—so side effects can occur throughout the body.

Women who have no signs of cancer in their

lymph nodes and women who have not gone through menopause will usually be given low doses of chemotherapy (anticancer drugs). Women who have cancer cells in their lymph nodes will get higher doses of chemotherapy. Chemotherapy works by poisoning the cancer cells, but it affects some normal cells, too, so there are side effects including hair loss, nausea, vomiting, and decreased numbers of cells made by the bone marrow (which increases a woman's risk of infection). Generally, chemotherapy is given by mouth or intravenously (into a vein) over the course of 3 to 6 months. The side effects almost always end when the course of treatment ends. There are differences of opinion regarding types of drugs to use, in what combinations, and in what dosages. Every case must be evaluated individually.

Before hormone therapy is offered, tests may be done to determine whether the cancer has estrogen and progesterone receptors. Having these receptors is a good sign: women with them are more likely to respond to hormone treatment and have an improved chance of survival. If a woman has this type of breast cancer, she will be offered a hormone, *tamoxifen*. It blocks the effects of estrogen on the breast and thus stops the growth of the cancer. The treatment may last for a number of years. Women treated with tamoxifen have a lower incidence of cancer in the other breast. Side effects include symptoms of menopause—hot flashes and vaginal dryness.

Some studies suggest that women who take tamoxifen have an increased risk of developing cancer in the lining of the uterus. For this reason, regular exams—and sometimes biopsies—of the lining of the uterus are usually done in women taking tamoxifen. There is now research being conducted to determine whether tamoxifen will prevent breast cancer in women who are at high risk but who have not yet been diagnosed with breast cancer.

Breast Reconstruction

If a woman has had a breast removed because of cancer, she may want to consider breast reconstruction. A woman contemplating reconstructive surgery needs to make several choices; the most obvious one is whether to have the surgery. Only 30 percent of women who have mastectomies choose breast reconstruction. This choice shouldn't affect how they choose to have their cancer treated, although desire for reconstruction should be discussed with the surgeon treating the cancer. The way cancer surgery is done can affect whether and how reconstruction is done. The decision-making process should involve not only the patient and her cancer surgeon but also the surgeon doing the reconstruction (a plastic and reconstructive surgeon).

Factors to consider in the decision about reconstructive surgery include the woman's medical condition and degree of tissue loss, the need for additional therapy, and her general health. Reconstruction can be more painful and difficult than the original cancer operation, so all factors should be carefully considered.

Psychological factors must be evaluated as well; some women feel that only reconstruction can put an end to the trauma of losing a breast. Women who choose reconstruction often experience profound improvement in their mental attitude afterward. But each woman will have to evaluate for herself whether reconstruction will help her get on with her life after breast cancer.

If a woman chooses not to have reconstructive surgery, she can use an external prosthesis (artificial breast) worn inside her clothing. A woman's appearance in clothes, as well as her level of physical activity, will influence how comfortable she'll be using a prosthesis.

If a woman chooses reconstructive surgery, it sometimes can be done at the same time as the surgery for cancer. Other times, it will be done in a later operation. Some of the types of procedures that may be done include the following:

- Insertion of a saline or silicone implant, often after tissue expansion (but note new FDA restrictions on silicone implants)
- Use of the woman's own muscles (taken from the back, abdomen, or buttock) to reconstruct the breast
- Reconstruction of the nipple and areola

Support for Women with Cancer

It's important that a woman who has breast cancer consider all the support services she can. A recent study showed that women who belonged to a support group had a higher rate of survival than women who had the same physical treatment but no support group. The American Cancer Society, the local hospital, physicians, and local therapists or counseling centers can help you find a support group. Some women are motivated to start a group. For many women this action not only helps them cope better but also may determine the extent of their physical recovery.

Diagnosis of Benign Lumps

To the touch, a cyst can feel like a solid lump, so much of the workup for a cyst will be the same as for a solid lump. Your doctor will take a history and examine you to confirm what you've found (if in fact you yourself have detected a problem). Be sure to tell the doctor exactly where the lump is located, how long it has been present, how big it is, if it has changed during your monthly cycle, and if it is tender.

If you are age 30 or older, mammography will usually be done. An ultrasound exam may be done to see whether the lump is fluid filled (a cyst) or solid. If a lump can be felt, it is usually better to have a fine needle aspiration. If the lump is a cyst, it will disappear as a consequence of the aspiration and is thereby treated at the same time it's diagnosed. No further treatment is required. Because so few cysts contain abnormal cells, it's not routine to send fluid for laboratory examination unless it is bloody, which might indicate cancer. If the lump doesn't go away following aspiration, a biopsy should be performed.

Cosmetic Surgery

The decision to have breast surgery to alter appearance is a very personal one, involving complex issues of self-esteem, body image, even personal empowerment. It's a decision a woman needs to make carefully.

Breasts can be either enlarged or reduced. For either type of surgery, a woman should get complete information from her doctor about how the procedure is done, the risks, and what type of final appearance to expect. Because breast enlargement is a cosmetic procedure done on healthy breasts, it is not usually covered by health insurance.

Breast Infections

The main symptom of breast infection is inflammation—redness and pain in the breast or any part of it. There are three possible causes.

- *Lactational mastitis.* This is a buildup of bacteria caused by a plugged milk duct in a woman who is breast-feeding. The diagnosis is usually based on the woman's history and physical exam findings; no special tests are needed.

  Treatment involves using hot compresses and hot showers in which the water is allowed to flow over the breast. If symptoms don't ease within 24 hours, antibiotics will be added. It's fine to continue nursing; neither the antibiotics nor the bacteria will harm the baby, and keeping the breasts emptied will ease the woman's discomfort.
- *Nonlactational mastitis.* Causes of this infection vary, but the symptoms resemble those of lactational mastitis. It is diagnosed and treated the same way.
- *Chronic subareolar abscess.* This is an uncommon infection in the oil glands around the nipple. It is difficult to treat; antibiotics may help, but usually surgical drainage becomes necessary. Since this is a chronic—or recurring—condition, the involved duct and tract are often

removed; sometimes all of the ducts have to be removed. Very rarely, the entire nipple and areola have to be removed to control the infection. A woman should not have a mastectomy for this condition unless all previous measures have failed.

Noncancerous Breast Lumps

Not every breast lump is a sign of cancer. There are three common types of benign (noncancerous) breast lumps.

- *Fibrocystic changes.* Many women who have not yet gone through menopause have occasional pain or overall lumpiness in their breasts. These changes are called *fibrocystic changes.* It is natural for breast tissue to change in degree of "lumpiness" throughout a woman's hormonal cycle and also as she ages. The female hormones estrogen and progesterone are thought to be somehow involved in fibrocystic changes, but the cause is not known for sure. The tissue usually returns to normal after menstruation. After menopause, women's breasts become smoother in texture. Because these changes are so common and so little is known about their cause, they are hard to treat and cannot really be cured. Treatments that have been used include vitamins and advice to stay away from caffeine and chocolate. None of these has been a complete success. Breast pain can be treated by wearing a well-fitting bra, using pain medication, and limiting fluids, especially before the menstrual period. Fibrocystic changes do not increase the risk of cancer.

- *Cyst.* This is a fluid-filled sac that usually occurs in women in their 40s and early 50s. It is caused by reabsorption of the breast lobules that occurs naturally as a woman approaches menopause. Cysts may be present on and off for several years; often they occur in groups. They are almost always harmless, but it is impossible to distinguish between a cyst or a solid breast mass simply by feeling it, so aspiration or a biopsy will usually be recommended.
- *Fibroadenoma.* This is a solid lump found mostly in women in their 20s and 30s. It results from excess formation of the lobules (milk-producing glands) and stroma (the connective tissue in the breast). The lump feels round and smooth, and often "shoots" to a different part of the breast when pushed upon. Such lumps are rarely cancerous, but usually should be biopsied just to be sure.

RESOURCES FOR MORE INFORMATION

The National Cancer Institute (NCI) is a good resource for information and publications about cancer-related subjects. Call the Cancer Information Service (800-4CANCER). The general public can receive information by fax as well; call 301-402-5874 from a touch-tone phone and follow the directions.

If a woman facing chemotherapy would like

more information about individual drugs, she can call the NCI at 800-422-6237 and ask for "Anticancer Drug Information Sheets" for her particular drug.

Another source of information is the American Cancer Society (800-ACS-2345).

PART III

Pain Evaluation and Management

Kathleen M. Foley, M.D.

The term *pain* is pervasive throughout our society, as shown in our common expressions, such as "a pain in the neck" or "no pain, no gain," both of which imply our negative feeling toward pain. Actually, pain can be positive or negative. On one hand, pain warns a person that there is something wrong with part of her body. On the other hand, chronic pain often serves no useful purpose, giving only lifelong trouble to the person dealing with it.

Long ago, pain was thought to be the body saying something was wrong with one of its physical parts. Now we know pain is not only physical, but also has mental components. The unique pain felt by a specific woman with an injury or disease depends on the situation, on the woman, and on her genetic makeup. No matter how individual each person's pain is, however, pain is a reality that causes many people discomfort, disturbance of sleep and appetite, and even depression.

WHAT IS PAIN?

Physical pain is a physiological response of the body to a stimulus. It occurs when any of the body's pain receptors has an internal or external physical reaction to a stimulus that activates the nerves. Pain is defined as an unpleasant sensory and emotional experience associated with the actual physical or potential tissue damage. This subjective experience cannot be measured in any quantifiable way. Psychological pain usually has no apparent injury or physiological explanation, even though the patient describes the symptoms in terms of physical hurt (see Table 3.1).

TABLE 3.1 COMMON SOURCES OF PAIN

Imbalances in the Body

Digestive (gastroenteritis, ulcers, irritable bowel syndrome, hemorrhoids, diverticulitis, gas, inflammatory bowel disease, appendicitis)

Urinary (bladder infection, kidney or ureteral stones)

Reproductive system (menstrual symptoms, menopause, pregnancy, fibroid tumors, ovarian cysts, endometriosis, cervical polyps)

Upper respiratory system (pneumonia, colds, flu)

Brain and nerves (aneurysm, thrombophlebitis, neuralgia)

Physical Injuries

Back (aches and disk)

Eyes (eyestrain, infections, pinkeye)

Ears (altitude-related ear pain, infection)

Face (TMD, neuralgia)

Hand and arm (carpal tunnel syndrome, bursitis, tendonitis, Raynaud's syndrome)

Leg and foot (bone spurs, corns and bunions, varicose veins, muscle cramps, thrombosis, ingrown toenails)

Nose and throat (sore throat, strep throat, sinusitis)

Teeth and gums (gingivitis, periodontitis, toothache, mouth sores)

Skin (frostbite and sunburn, fire burns)

Pain from Disease

Contagious diseases (mumps, chicken pox, shingles, measles)

Degenerative diseases (bones and joints—arthritis, osteoporosis, gout)

Sexually transmitted diseases (herpes, AIDS, pelvic inflammatory disease)

Other disease (diabetes, cancer, heart disease, sickle cell anemia)

How We Feel Pain

The feeling of pain occurs when nerve endings detect damage to the body. These free nerve endings, or pain receptors (nociceptors), sense the changes in the body that are translated in the brain as pain. Pain receptors respond to three conditions: pressure, such as hammering a finger; heat, such as burning an arm; and chemical changes around the nerve endings, such as prostaglandins, chemicals released by damaged cells.

Pain-generating nerve endings are in the skin, organs, muscles, joints, and tendons; they can be external or internal. External pain is caused by outside influences, such as cutting a finger or stubbing a toe; internal pain may be more disturbing, as the stimulus—and often the hurting internal organ, muscle, or bone—cannot be seen. Headaches and migraines are examples. Pain originating in visceral or internal organs is not well understood, as they can be cut, burned, or crushed without any pain to the patient; yet chemical burns, spasms, and ischemia (tissue anemia) can provoke intense pain in certain organs. Not all pain comes as the result of a direct stimulus—indirect problems from pain are also possible. For example, an arthritis victim may walk in a different way because of pain, thus causing another type of pain unlike the change in walking patterns.

When you feel pain, certain reactions take place in less than a second. Nerve fibers carry chemical signals from the pain receptors to a specific area of the spinal cord: C nerve fibers signal slow, burning, aching, and long-term pain, such as the residual ache from a burned finger, or the chronic pain from cancer. Thick, A-delta nerve fibers signal faster, more localized or acute pain; these are responsible for our faster pain-induced reactions, such as instantly removing a hand from a hot stove.

Fibers from other sections of the body join at certain sites along the spinal cord, and from there, fiber bundles, or tracts, carry the pain messages to the brain stem cortex. Even as the pain signal is sent to the cortex, other information is sent from the spinal cord to various parts of the brain controlling specific parts of the body. The heart rate and blood pressure may increase, breathing increases, and the pupils dilate; adrenaline and sugar may rush into the bloodstream to increase energy to prepare the body for the possible stress of pain. When the nerve signals reach the thalamus, deep in the middle of the brain, they are translated to indicate where the pain is and what type of pain it is. At the same time, signals are sent back down to the spinal cord to modulate the sensation of pain, thus raising our threshold of pain.

The overall nervous system has many overlapping and redundant features, such as densely packed pain receptors that deliver information to the brain and other parts of the body when pain is felt. This is an indication that pain is a primitive sense, built into our systems to allow us to better survive. Too much pain would disable us. Conversely, having no nerves to detect and deliver pain information would threaten our survival as we would not be aware of trauma or infections.

Anxiety and Pain

There is a direct connection between pain and anxiety, an emotion that accompanies most feelings of pain. Most of the time, we experience little anxiety with familiar types of pain, especially a hurt that can be easily explained such as sunburn or banging the head on an open cabinet door. We feel more anxiety when we do not understand the pain or when it is excessive, such as sudden excessive painful aches in the head or abdomen.

Such pain leads to worries about dreaded diseases or incurable pain; and these thoughts cause the body to react: the pulse quickens; breathing, heart rate, and sweating increase; and muscles become tense. Often such a reaction worsens the feeling of pain, causing the person to perceive that she is experiencing even more pain. Studies have shown that such excessive anxiety also can affect the recovery of a patient undergoing surgery for a painful physical ailment. A patient with less anxiety going into surgery recovers faster and has less pain associated with the surgery than one who is anxiety-ridden before surgery.

Chest Pains

Contrary to popular belief, chest pains have a variety of causes. Anxiety causes some chest pains, most often from the quicker intake of breaths during times of such stress. We normally breathe about 14 to 16 times per minute; when anxiety strikes, our breaths become shallow and almost double in number. Thus, less oxygen can reach our chest muscles and help them work. This results in a tenderness around the cartilage connecting the ribs and the breastbone. Colds (upper respiratory infections) or pneumonia can cause chest discomfort, especially from excessive coughing.

Also, chest pain may originate from angina pectoris, or a pressure in the chest that comes and goes, usually during physical activity or emotional stress when the heart needs more oxygen-rich blood than it receives. The lack of oxygen—most often caused by a plaque partially blocking the walls of arteries leading to the heart—can cause a constricting chest pain that can spread to the jaw, neck, and arms. It usually lasts less than 10 minutes. Most angina patients have prescriptions, including nitroglycerin tablets that open up constricted blood vessels, to alleviate the pain of angina.

The chest pain associated with a heart attack feels like a pressure in the chest that can range from mild to unbearable. The signs and symptoms of a heart attack include breathing difficulty and sweating. The pulse may be fast, slow, or irregular, while the victim is pale or bluish in color. The overall symptoms that indicate a heart attack are usually associated with pains in the shoulder and down the left arm or to the jaw.

Childbirth and Pain

Most women experience pain with contractions during childbirth, with the peak intensity of pain between the time when the cervix opening is fully dilated and contractions in the uterus push the baby into the vagina and out of the body. During labor, there are several ways to reduce the pain:

Change your position by adopting an upright position, kneeling on all fours, or squatting. Breathe slowly and rhythmically to help you relax. Narcotics, usually used to help the mother relax, are commonly administered in the middle of labor but not at the last part of labor, as they may cause the baby to have difficulty breathing. Local anesthesia is used for a forceps delivery or episiotomy. General anesthesia usually is used if a Cesarean section is warranted.

Epidural anesthesia, an anesthetic drug injected into the spine, numbs the mother from the waist down when other pain-relieving measures during labor pain do not work. This anesthesia generally wears off when the baby is being delivered, so the mother can still push the baby effectively. The issue of using drugs during childbirth to reduce pain is highly debated. Several issues are involved, including the rights of the mother to experience the birth without clouding her thinking; the ease of delivery with or without drugs; and the effects the drugs will have on the baby. And there are trade-offs to all the aspects of drugs and childbirth. For example, early in labor drugs to control vomiting are administered in case narcotics or anesthesia must be given later due to an emergency; these may alter the mother's awareness. Local anesthetics are frequently used, which leave the mother's mind clear but partially paralyze the lumbar area; this weakens the contractions and slows down the labor.

What are the best alternatives to using drugs to ease the pain of childbirth? Although it does not appeal to everyone, many women choose to use prepared childbirth training. Such training includes the Lamaze training that prepares the mother so she knows what to expect and decreases the anxiety that can increase her pain. It features relaxation training to help the mother calm herself when the contractions increase in number and intensity; using techniques to distract attention from the pain; and breathing exercises to help relax and aid in the birthing process.

NATURAL PAIN RELIEF

The delicate balance between our perception of too much or not much pain is controlled by chemicals produced naturally within our body. This special system helps the body to deal with stress and pain. A chemical called substance P is thought to be important in transmitting the pain signals from the skin to the spinal cord. Thus, people who are insensitive to pain are thought to be deficit in substance P. The body also produces at least eight naturally occurring opiates, including endorphins and enkephalins. All are more powerful than any opiates derived from plants such as opium.

Natural opiates are molecules of pain-suppressing chemicals also called neurotransmitters; they transmit information among and between the roughly 100 billion cells (neurons) in the brain. The neurons fire electrical chemical impulses at varying rates, triggering the release of the neurotransmitters and causing other nerve cells to fire. In the nervous systems of most vertebrate animals, the natural painkillers (also called neurochemicals or opiate peptides) endorphin and enkephalin interact with some nerve cells on sites called opiate receptors (as do opiate drugs such as morphine). When the painkillers bind with the opiate receptors, usually at an area of gray matter surrounding a fluid-filled canal in the brain, they modulate the nerve impulses across the nerve synapses, reducing or relieving pain.

Natural Highs

The opiate peptides called endorphins are present throughout the brain and appear to control pain principally at the brain stem. Enkephalins act mainly within the spinal cord where this natural painkiller blocks the transmission of pain signals. Researchers studying why the synthetic painkiller morphine affects the body eventually discovered the body's endorphins in 1975. *Endorphin* is a contraction of "endogenously manufactured morphinelike substance," or a morphinelike chemical manufactured by the body.

Researchers have connected the release of endorphins to many other body functions and responses; they believe endorphins significantly alter the body's blood cholesterol levels (in reaction to stress), memory, learning, sexual activity, depression, and schizophrenia. A well-known effect of endorphins (in particular, beta-endorphins) occurs after vigorous aerobic exercise. Also known as a runner's high, the release of endorphins occurs after about 12 minutes of strenuous workout. This may be the body's way of coping with the pain of exercise—by raising its resistance to pain.

Beta-endorphins are uniquely different than the other opiate peptides found in several regions of the brain. Beta-endorphins occur only in cells around the brain's highest levels and in the pituitary gland, which releases beta-endorphins at the same time it releases ACTH, a stress hormone. During World War II, wounded soldiers required fewer painkillers than civilians undergoing elective surgery; even though the soldiers were subjected to terrible battle wounds, the stress of combat increased the amount of endorphins, and thus ACTH, altering the soldiers' perception of pain.

HOW TO COMMUNICATE WITH YOUR PHYSICIAN ABOUT YOUR PAIN

The most common way to describe pain to your health care provider is by using her terminology:

- *Generalized pain* is a hurt felt all over the body with no real specific central location, such as certain pains from cancer.
- *Local pain* is a hurt in one specific region, such as a broken finger.
- *Referred pain* is a hurt felt at a site that is at a distance from the injury or diseased part. For example, a toothache may be referred to the ear, because they share the same sensory nerves; angina, a chest pain caused by a reduction in blood supply to the heart, often is felt in the left arm or shoulder. Even an injury in the knee can be felt in the hip area.
- *Acute pain* is a response to some physical ailment or stimulus of sudden onset. It usually occurs as an injury, such as the hammering of a finger, or as the result of a previous and continual exposure to a pain-causing stimulus, such as a sunburn or postoperative pain. An attack of appendicitis or kidney stones can cause acute pain. Most acute pain can be a warning signal that something is wrong and that to avoid further damage you should seek medical attention. Some injuries cause a delayed or subacute pain,

such as whiplash that is felt hours or days after an accident.

- *Chronic pain* occurs as a symptom to an underlying disease or problem. It usually lasts more than 3 months. Chronic pain often develops gradually, such as a back or shoulder ache, or arthritis. After an injury or disease is cured, chronic pain can still persist, often due to permanent nerve damage or scar tissue buildup. Chronic pain can be barely noticeable to debilitating; it can vary as to the times it strikes—ranging from constant, or minute to minute, to every other day. *Chronic pain syndrome* causes changes in a person, including physical problems (sleep and appetite disturbance, fatigue), psychological problems (irritability, depression), family problems, and social withdrawal.

There are several additional ways to talk with a doctor about your pain: If you know the source of your pain, such as a bee sting, or recurrent sinus infection, explain to your doctor what happened or prior occurrences of a certain pain. This helps the doctor pinpoint how to treat your pain. Be specific about your pain: describe its timing, nature, location, severity, or if it radiates from one spot.

Note if the pain occurs at certain times during the day (such as after you eat or when you exercise), if any foods trigger the pain (such as shellfish or milk products), or if you have had the same pain in the past.

Pain is the most common symptom causing patients to seek medical attention. Not everyone responds in the same way to pain, making it a highly individual experience. Even two people feeling pain from the exact same stimulus and under similar conditions feel their pain in different ways. Commonly, these two people would define their pain differently, even though they are experiencing the same disease or stimuli. This is why methods to relieve pain may work for one person but not work for the next.

Realize that there may not be a cure for your pain. Some types of pain go on indefinitely and it is necessary to live with such pain. When you need relief from chronic pain, ask your doctor to help you manage your pain or to refer you to a pain clinic or specialty group that can help you to understand and better cope with the pain.

CHOICES IN THE MANAGEMENT OF PAIN

Patients have numerous choices to eliminate or reduce acute or chronic pain under certain conditions. The most common approaches include (1) pain relievers that alter the body chemistry, and (2) physical, psychological, cognitive, anesthetic, and neurosurgical methods. No one can tell you the best method to relieve pain from your body; you must weigh the risks and benefits of various approaches. With your physician's help, you can tailor a treatment approach for your body and circumstances.

Drug Therapy

The most frequently used approach—mainly because it is fast and most in demand—is drug therapy. Even so, drug therapy is not always the safest way to eliminate pain; certain drugs can have side effects. Consult your physician before taking any medication; when a physician prescribes a medication for pain, ask about the possible side effects. Drug therapy utilizes anti-inflammatory drugs, narcotics, and antidepressants.

Anti-Inflammatory Drugs

The three types of anti-inflammatory drugs are corticosteroids, nonsteroidal anti-inflammatory drugs, and analgesics (although not all analgesics block pain). All three drugs also are used for other purposes. Most anti-inflammatory drugs are pain relievers to take care of the redness and burning associated with inflammation and help relieve general pain.

Corticosteroids

Corticosteroids are made from synthetic hormones and are used as anti-inflammatories, bronchodilators for asthma, and immunosuppressives.

Nonsteroidal Anti-Inflammatory Drugs

Nonsteroidal anti-inflammatory drugs (NSAID) include more than 20 substances and work by blocking the production of prostaglandins. These drugs are effective against slow, prolonged tissue damage and the associated pain, such as in the socket of an extracted tooth or arthritic joint, and general or localized pains, such as back pain, menstrual cramps, and headaches. NSAIDs are not effective against pain triggered by events that do not produce inflammatory reactions.

Analgesics

Analgesics include simple analgesics, such as aspirin and acetaminophen, for mild pain and narcotic analgesics, such as codeine and morphine, for severe pain. Analgesics such as aspirin work by reducing inflammation. They also prevent the production of prostaglandins, chemicals that the body produces when tissue is damaged (these chemicals combine with the opiate receptors on the surface of cells in the brain and spinal cord). Acetaminophens are the only analgesics that work by blocking pain impulses in the brain and preventing the perception of pain.

For patients with moderate to severe pain, doctors often combine narcotic analgesics with non-narcotic drugs. These include drugs such as hydrocodone, codeine, and propoxyphene that are useful for moderate pain often associated with mild trauma, headache, toothache, or backache. For patients suffering severe pain, the strong narcotic analgesics are useful; these include morphine, hydromorphine, and methadone. Doctors use this class of drugs most commonly to help patients manage acute postoperative pain and the severe chronic pain of cancer. Narcotic analgesics work by binding to the opiate receptors on the peripheral nerve as well as the central nervous system. Patients need to be aware that all of these analgesic drugs have side effects.

Local anesthetics are locally applied analgesics used for reducing pain; they include bupivacaine and lidocaine, which can be injected to deaden the nerve so pain is not felt during a dental procedure.

Doctors use local anesthetics to facilitate treatment of skin wounds and to numb areas of the body before surgery.

Narcotics

Narcotics are opiate drugs that block pain signals and inhibit the patient's perception of pain. Doctors use narcotics when pain is short-term and intense, such as with kidney stones, severe burns or injury, heart attacks, or after surgery. Narcotics are prescribed for chronic pain, only if other drug or nondrug therapies do not relieve the pain. In most cases, the dosage is such that the pain is brought to a bearable level so the patient can still mentally function.

Antidepressants

People who suffer from pain, especially chronic pain, often become depressed and are prescribed antidepressants. Low doses of such drugs can have an effect on pain. For example, low doses of mood-elevating drugs called tricyclic antidepressants seem to block pain messages traveling to the spinal cord or may change the way the nerve acts at the injury site. These antidepressants work best for nerve damage pain (such as diabetes, injuries, amputation, or viral infections that attack the nerves, like shingles); they include doxepin, amitriptyline, imipramine, and desipramine.

Regardless of the drug approach you and your doctor choose, it must be individualized for your pain problem. This includes the choice of drug, the way it is administered, and the time frame for its use.

Nondrug Techniques

Some nondrug techniques are just as good for certain pain reduction problems as drug therapy; often they carry less risk to the patient than medications. The success rate of such ministrations varies; it is up to the patient, with the help of the doctor and other experts, to determine the best treatment. They must consider the nature, site, and intensity of the pain. Most commonly, doctors combine drug and nondrug approaches to provide patients with comprehensive treatment.

Heat

One of the most ancient ways to decrease pain is to use heating techniques; no one knows why heat makes pain decrease. It is doubtful that heat speeds up repair of an injury. However, locally applied heat using simple methods such as heating pads, moist heat, and hot water bottles does reduce low to moderate levels of pain due to such injuries as bruises, torn muscles, and arthritis, and such pains as menstrual cramps or backaches. Ultrasound raises the temperature in deep structures under the skin to treat pain in joints or bones.

Cold

Another ancient technique to decrease pain is to use cold that constricts local blood vessels and makes the area feel numb. Researchers believe that the cold acts similar to acupuncture by producing a burning pain that may block pain signals. Ice has been used to decrease dental pain by massaging an ice cube on the back of the hand between the thumb and index finger. Ice also relieves the pain and swelling from sprains, bumps, and subsequent bruises.

TENS

The transcutaneous (across the skin) electrical nerve stimulation units (TENS) are available only through prescription. TENS units send a small electrical current pulse—less than 10 percent of a 60-watt lightbulb—that stimulates the nerve fibers just under the skin, blocking pain signals along the nerves. TENS units are used for just about every type of pain: wound pain; nerve injuries; face, mouth, and tooth pain; diametric nerve damage; cancer pain, itching; postoperative pain; labor pain; arthritis; headaches; and so on. The unit, about the size of a television remote control, is worn on the belt; the patient places the electrodes carrying the current at the site of the pain or over the acupuncture point near the pain. The pain is relieved while the unit is turned on or a short time after it is turned off. Many patients report that after over a year of use, the TENS unit loses its therapeutic abilities; apparently the nerve system begins to ignore the electrical stimulation and allows pain signals to break through.

Behavioral Techniques

Behavioral techniques that relieve pain use the mind to modify or eliminate pain, especially chronic pain. Although not for everyone, behavioral pain relief methods can replace medication; they should be taught in a professional facility by therapists who can provide advice and assistance.

Biofeedback

Feedback is a word taken from electronics that means information in a loop that is recorded and fed back into the system to adjust the operation. Biofeedback is similar, using the mind to control the body when tension is the cause of pain, rather than arthritis, cancer, or nerve damage. After being attached to sensors that monitor body readings, patients are able to see or hear muscle tension, temperature, and other body processes. With practice, patients eventually gain enough control over the process to change what they see or hear on the monitors. For example, temperature biofeedback is used for the treatment of migraine headaches; the temperature sensors show that as blood vessels narrow, body temperatures decrease. Patients learn to increase the blood flow to these areas with biofeedback; thus, by controlling their thinking they can decrease the occurrence of painful migraines.

Visualization

Visualization is a mental technique similar to biofeedback. Athletes use visualization to enhance their performance; over and over they see in their minds the perfect pitch, or precise pole jump. Visualization does not necessarily have to be in the mind; patients also can draw their illnesses, using the images to get rid of their pain or illness on paper. One type of visualization called guided imagery gives the patient a visual goal to accomplish, such as picturing being free of pain, or visualizing an image of a shrinking tumor. The patient is trained to ignore the pain by evoking imagery that is incompatible with the pain. Researchers believe that such visualization techniques cause the body to become less stressed.

Relaxation

Relaxation is the release of stress, anxiety, and often pain. Relaxation techniques include deep breathing, muscle relaxation techniques, and meditation. One of the best ways to relax is to meditate: Sit or lie down in a comfortable position, deeply relaxing all your muscles. Breathe at a relaxed rate through the nose, releasing all thoughts from your brain. Some people repeat one word over and over, focusing their attention on that word. This is usually done for about 20 minutes; however, there is no real set time to use relaxation techniques. Each individual develops her own rhythm of relaxation.

Hypnosis

Pain patients often turn to hypnosis; by using this form of relaxation they can shut out distraction and focus intensely on one particular subject, such as getting rid of pain. Not everyone is a candidate for hypnosis, because patients must be receptive to suggestion. After the diagnosis of a pain problem, hypnosis can be used as a potential alternative to treat the pain. It is used mainly for chronic pains, such as recurring headaches; or for relaxation, such as helping a woman to relax and thus experience less pain during labor.

Physical Techniques and Specialists

Exercise

Exercise is thought to relieve pain by forcing a patient to concentrate on something other than the pain; in addition, vigorous exercise causes the body to release natural painkillers into the bloodstream, thus decreasing pain. Exercise such as running, walking, skiing, biking, and hiking increase cardiovascular and overall endurance. Weight training increases muscular strength and decreases the chance of painful injuries, because the body is in shape. Exercise can include some of the more gentle motions that benefit organs and internal body structure. Some yoga instructors also include deep breathing and meditation with more traditional yoga exercises.

Massage

At one time or another, we have all rubbed a sore shoulder, or stretched an aching hamstring muscle to relieve pain. For deeper pains such as backaches, highly trained professionals use techniques that apply mechanical pressure to relieve the pain. There are many massage techniques; some massage the area of pain, while others use pressure on various parts of the body to relieve the pain.

Physical Therapy

Physical therapists are trained professionals who treat the musculoskeletal system; they cannot diagnose medical problems or prescribe medication. They use their hands and technology to treat a wide variety of pain problems, including cancer, strained or sprained muscles, and lower back pain. They customize each treatment, using techniques such as exercise programs, ultrasound, massage, and heat and cold applications.

Physiatry

Physiatrists are medical doctors who use physical methods and agents to treat patients, including those suffering pain. They can evaluate and prescribe treatment regimens for disabilities due to pain. Physical medicine emphasizes rehabilitation and uses other health care professionals in a team approach to diagnose and relieve pain.

Alternative Health Techniques

Alternative health methods provide an alternative to drugs and drug therapy; they use numerous healing techniques to relieve pain.

Acupuncture

Acupuncture, the ancient Chinese healing art, uses various therapeutic techniques, including the insertion of various-size needles at specific points on the body called meridians. Classic texts describe 365 acupuncture points, each associated with specific organs. According to acupuncturists, the needles allow the body to flow; they are used to maintain health or eliminate imbalances in the body, including the relief of pain. Researchers believe that acupuncture may work because the stimulating needles cause the release of endorphins, thus lessening pain or giving the patient a feeling of well-being.

Acupressure

Very similar to acupuncture, acupressure is a method of using pressure to work on the meridians of the body to treat specific pain symptoms or disorders.

Hydrotherapy

Hydrotherapy uses water to relieve the constant pressures on certain parts of the body and reduce pain. The most common types of treatment are swimming and water exercises, usually for chronic back problems.

Surgery

Surgery to relieve pain often is a last resort. It may seem as if just cutting a nerve will cause the feeling of pain to disappear. In reality, cutting nerves to cut pain usually leads to other complications, such as numbness. Nerve blocks to temporarily deaden neural pathways that conduct pain also have been used to control pain; they leave the area insensitive to a pinprick. Chronic pain patients report the pain still persists even though the area is numb.

The following neurosurgical approaches have been tried to relieve pain, but there have been very few successes. Pain often returns in a different place or is more intense than before surgery.

- The patient's sympathetic system can be surgically or chemically destroyed; the sympathetic system supplies the blood vessels and glands, and affects blood flow and pressure. This operation is difficult and usually does not relieve pain.
- A cordotomy involves cutting the tracts in the spinal cord. This usually cuts the paths to the spinal cord, and disrupts signals to the thalamus; there are so many nerve fibers destined for the thalamus that it is a difficult operation. The major problem is that the effect fades as months go by.
- Cerebral (brain) operations have been used in the past, directly targeting the pain centers even though the true sites of pain are still not known; these operations have very few successes.

Psychological Help

Pain does not always follow physiological paths—the patient's mental state also has a direct effect on her perception of pain. In many cases, part of an injured patient's stress is emotional distress as well as the awareness of physical injury. During childbirth, or after surgery, emotional distress may be a major aspect of the patient's pain. Research has shown that the intensity and duration of pain for postoperative patients has a direct relationship to the patient's psychological preparation before the operation by counselors and the physician's explanation of the operation.

Because of this direct link between pain and emotion, doctors realize that some patients' pain, especially chronic pain, may be helped using psychological approaches. In fact, psychological pain usually cannot be treated physiologically. The psychologists try to understand how much of the patient's pain is due to psychological factors, such as depression, or job or family difficulties. They work with patients' families to increase their awareness of the patients' pain and to decrease factors in the home that may contribute to their pain. For patients who are thinking too much about the pain—concentrating so hard on the pain that it is more overwhelming than reality—psychologists help them overcome such feelings.

Psychologists also look at patients' pain in terms of behavior: Are they getting out of a stressful situation by using their pain as an excuse? Are they getting attention because of pain? Another situation often occurs: Even if they have had the pain for months or years, patients are in a constant state of alarm, believ-

IS IT ALL IN MY HEAD?

One of the main questions for those suffering from chronic pain is whether the pain is all in their heads. This question usually is asked about long-term pain or when no real diagnosis for the pain has been made. Pain almost always has a real physical basis; only about 5 percent of chronic pain is psychological rather than physical.

Patients who experience psychogenic or psychological pain do so for two major reasons: They have hallucinations (or a false perception of reality) or delusions (usually depressed patients have a false belief relating to their bodies). Less frequent reasons include conversion reactions in which sensations (such as the complaint of a pain) are compensating for some intense emotion; and hypochondriasis, in which the patient has a fascination with the experience of illness.

ing there is really something else wrong. As such anxiety continues, patients become worse; their fears are confirmed by a self-fulfilling prophecy.

Most psychological situations involving pain can be helped by psychological techniques. Psychologists use such techniques as having patients make goals for themselves; positive thinking; tuning out the pain; and helping patients answer hard questions about their pain. Another way patients can cope with pain is by attending group therapy sessions; often these include patients who are trying to cope with the same types of pain.

GETTING HELP

Patients who experience pain—either chronic or acute—are not alone. Pain clinics and organizations can help them understand their options, including how to talk about, understand, and cope with the pain. For a person in chronic pain, this can be the difference between living a fulfilling life or existing in a debilitating situation.

Often pain patients are advised to set goals for themselves; working toward their goals gives them a feeling of accomplishment. The goals should be the antitheses of pain, such as setting goals at work (even if it means changing careers), taking classes for enjoyment, or actively working so many hours or minutes a day in the garden (even with adaptations to make it easier).

The pain patient should be realistic about her pain. For example, a patient with degenerative joint problems must be realistic about the chronic pain, and understand that when all the alternative cures or treatments are exhausted she must live with the pain. This is probably the most difficult step of all, but it is most important in coping with chronic pain.

Pain patients are encouraged to become as active as they can in their work, recreation, and social activities. It does no good to ignore the mental and physical health benefits of being active in all aspects of their lives. Pain patients are encouraged to talk with others about their hurt—especially other pain patients—and continue optimistically with life.

There are numerous pain clinics across the country. When looking for a pain clinic, keep the following points in mind:

- Make sure the program is legitimate; pain centers that are part of hospitals or rehabilitation centers usually offer a more comprehensive treatment than stand-alone clinics.
- The program should have several types of professionals on staff, including physicians (neurologist, psychiatrist, physiatrist, or anesthesiologist with expertise in pain management), registered nurse, physical therapist, biofeedback therapist, vocational counselor, family counselor, personnel trained in pain management intervention, and occupational therapist.
- Patients should look for a program that is convenient for them and their families to attend; they should make sure that their families can be included in their pain care. The facility should be close enough to enable patients to comfortably commute every day or as often as their programs demand.
- Patients should examine the clinic to see if it has the following features: biofeedback, relaxation, and stress management training, counseling (individual and family), TENS unit, physical therapy, educational program (explaining medications and pain management), group and occupational therapy, assertiveness training, and aftercare.

Other patient concerns when selecting a clinic include: what your insurance company covers; whether the program is part of a hospital; what will be required of you during your stay (including what you should bring with you); does the clinic have all your previous medical records, including allergies;

can you interview past and present patients at the clinic to learn about their experience at the clinic.

Pain Organizations

To discover which pain clinics are closest or best for you, contact one of the following organizations. You may also want to join some of the groups, as they often offer newsletters or booklets on coping with pain.

1. Commission on Accreditation of Rehabilitation Facilities (800-444-8991)
2. The American Chronic Pain Association (916-632-0922)
3. American Pain Society (708-966-5595)
4. The American Academy of Physical Medicine and Rehabilitation (312-922-9366)
5. The Chronic Pain Support Group (216-657-2948)
6. National Committee on the Treatment of Intractable Pain (301-983-1710)

PART IV

Managing Medication

Jean A. Hamilton, M.D., and
Kimberly A. Yonkers, M.D.

More than half of all visits to a doctor result in at least one prescription, and over a lifetime women make more visits than men. Women will likely be prescribed more drugs than the average man. Yet, until recently many new medications were tested and studied more extensively in men. Doctors know much less about how medication use affects their prime recipients, women.

It is known, however, that the sexes respond differently to certain kinds of medicines. Their bodies may process the medication differently, and they may experience beneficial or negative side effects. Some of these variations are related to the differences in body type between men and women. But women experience many physiological and psychological changes in their lives; the way women respond to medicines may alter as they go through menstruation, pregnancy, menopause, and aging.

Many doctors prescribing medications today were educated before all this new information was understood and accepted. Some still have a paternalistic attitude toward women and their health concerns. Thus, many doctors are playing catch-up, prescribing medications with an imagined male model patient in mind, whether or not the real patient is a woman or a man. When you realize the special sex-related issues of medication, both you and your doctor benefit from a better knowledge of how a particular medication is likely to affect you, the real patient. But first you have to understand how medications work in the body.

A QUICK COURSE IN PHARMACOLOGY

Pharmacology is the study of medications. *Pharmacotherapy* refers to the practice of using medications for therapeutic or preventive purposes. Because some groups of people respond differently to a given medication than do others, the goal of research is increasingly to make drug treatments work for members of various groups. Optimizing medication use for women is part of a larger, positive trend.

How Medications Work

How well medications work in the body depends on many factors. These factors can be simplified to the following four main steps needed for safe, effective medication use:

1. The medication must be *absorbed* into the body.
2. The medication must be *distributed* to the place in the body where it's needed.
3. The medication must be *metabolized* (broken down into parts) so that dangerously high levels do not build up.
4. Unabsorbed medication and broken-down medication must be *eliminated* from the body.

Any factor that affects how a medication is absorbed, distributed, metabolized, or eliminated affects the safety and effectiveness of the medication.

Absorption

The absorption of a medication into the body is determined by the health of the body, the type of medication, and the route by which the medication is taken. Many medications taken by mouth are digested in the intestines, where they are passed into the bloodstream. For these medications to be properly absorbed, the intestines need to be functioning normally. If not, much of the medication may pass uselessly out of the body.

The type of medication plays a role, too. Some types are more readily absorbed in an empty stomach; others enter the body faster when taken with food. Pills with coatings to protect the stomach from irritation have to be broken down in the intestines, so they are absorbed more slowly than pills without such a coating. Some medications can enter the body more readily through the membranes of the mouth, and get into the bloodstream quickly. This method is particularly useful for medications like nitroglycerin, which is used to relieve the chest pains of angina, a condition of decreased blood supply to the heart.

Distribution

Once medications have been absorbed into the bloodstream, they must be distributed to the place in the body where they're most needed. The size and composition of the body—the amount of blood and fluids and the percentage of muscle versus fatty tissue—affect distribution. Some medications are more likely to be stored in fatty tissue than others.

Metabolism

To prevent toxic, or dangerous, levels of medications from building up, the body has to find a way to break down the medication. This happens through a process called *metabolism.* Generally the metabolic process is done by enzymes, special types of proteins that act to break down or bind drugs to other substances. The metabolites, products that result from metabolism, may be "active," have a drug effect, or they may be inert.

Medications that pass from the stomach and intestines into the bloodstream first stop off in the liver. There, the liver gets a chance to metabolize the medicine before it gets into the general bloodstream and spreads throughout the body. With repeated circulation more and more of the drug is broken down by the liver. So, a healthy liver is a must for the proper metabolism of medications.

You need the right enzymes to break down the medication, too. Your genes and chromosomes, the body's blueprint, control the production of enzymes. Some women may inherit a blueprint in which an enzyme is absent or present in subnormal amounts. If this happens, the rate at which the body can break down certain medications slows.

Sometimes, one medication will speed up metabolic activity in the liver. This may cause other medications to be broken down faster, leading to lower levels of the drug in the body. These lower levels are less effective and so higher doses are needed. In this way, *tolerance* to medications occurs. Tolerance is particularly a problem with medications that can be abused, such as narcotics (heroin, morphine), sleeping pills (barbiturates), depressants (alcohol), and stimulants (amphetamines, caffeine, nicotine).

Elimination

Medications that have not been absorbed by the body and the elements resulting from the process of metabolism need a way to exit the body. As might be expected, most medications are mainly eliminated either through the liver into the bile to the feces or into the urine. Disturbances in the digestive system or urinary tract can affect how this occurs, however. If you have diarrhea, for example, food and medications rush through your digestive tract without getting a chance to be absorbed. The amount of medication you eliminate might be higher than normal and not enough of the medication would be available for use by your body. If there is a blockage to the biliary system in the liver, medications would not be eliminated by this route. In the urinary tract, kidney function can affect whether drugs and their metabolites are eliminated rapidly or slowly. If kidney function is significantly decreased, the dosage of drugs eliminated by this route must be decreased.

There are other routes out of the body, though, and some amounts of many medications can be found in tears, sweat, and saliva. Women who are breast-feeding can excrete some medications in their breast milk. Breast-feeding women should always consult their obstetrician or pediatrician before taking such medication.

Measures of Effectiveness in Medication

Pharmacologists and doctors often summarize the activity of medications in terms such as:

- *Bioavailability.* The amount of medication that the body can actually use.
- *Blood levels.* The amount of medication in the blood, which is related to the effectiveness (or efficacy) of the drug and its side effects.

- *Clearance.* The removal of a medication from the body.
- *Half-life.* The amount of time it takes for half of the medication to be eliminated from the body.

Bioavailability

One of the ways doctors compare the effectiveness of a medication is bioavailability. Not all of an ingested medication reaches its target. Some is eliminated without being used. When a medication has good bioavailability, it means that more of the medication is available for use. If the bioavailability is poor, less of the medication can be used, so more must be taken.

A similar measure of medication effectiveness is potency. Potency refers to the effectiveness in relation to the amount of drugs used. Less medication is needed if it has high potency, while more is needed if it is low.

Blood Levels

Once medication is absorbed into the bloodstream, its concentration in the blood can be measured. This is very helpful to doctors in determining how well the medication is working. If the blood levels are too low—which is known as low efficacy—the medication will not produce an adequate effect. If the blood levels of medication are too high, the risks for toxicity and side effects increase. Some side effects are just a nuisance, but others can be serious or even life threatening. Toxicity refers to a situation in which high levels of a drug can become dangerous, like a poison rather than a helpful medication.

Clearance

Clearance, or the removal of a medication from the body, can also be measured. If clearance is slower than normal, the medication can build up to dangerous levels. If clearance is faster than normal, the medication may be eliminated from the body before it has had a chance to act.

Half-Life

A medication's half-life refers to the amount of time it takes for one-half of the medication to be broken down in the body or eliminated. Medications with short half-lives are only active for hours; those with a long half-life are active for days. Half-life dictates dosing schedules—whether a drug is taken several times daily or once daily. Some medicines are specially treated with coatings that make them "slow releasing (SR)," so that they can be taken only once daily.

HOW SEX DIFFERENCES AFFECT MEDICATIONS

Many medications are processed differently by men and women, although a greater number *do not* show sex differences. (See Table 4.1)

When sex differences are noted, women tend to show *greater bioavailability*—that is, more of the medication is available for use. They also display *slower apparent clearance*—the slower elimination of the medication from the body—compared with

TABLE 4.1. SAMPLE OF MEDICATIONS THAT DO NOT SHOW SEX DIFFERENCES

Medication	Reason Used
Acebutolol	Lowers high blood pressure
Bupropion*	An antidepressant
Caffeine†	A stimulant found in coffee, tea, and some painkilling medications
Cimetidine	Suppresses stomach acid production; used in treating ulcers
Clonazepam	Prevents and treats seizures
Metoprolol	Treats high blood pressure
Phenytoin†	Prevents or treats seizures
Theophylline	Opens the blood vessels; used to treat asthma and other breathing problems, also stimulates the heart
Triazolam	A tranquilizer

*Although buproprion does not show sex differences, a person with the eating disorder bulimia is more likely to have seizures when taking this medication. Bulimia is much more common in girls and women than in men.

†This medication may be affected by hormones, either those naturally found in the body or those taken as medication (for example, birth control pills).

men. These sex-related differences suggest that the standard dose for a medication (probably based on studies of men) may be fairly high for women. Unless your doctor adjusts the dosage of a medication, your risk of having side effects or building up dangerous levels of the medication is higher. In fact, women tend to have side effects from medications about twice as often as men. (See Table 4.2 for some examples of sex differences in medications.) Researchers believe that medications that affect the brain and behavior (the psychotropic drugs) are more likely to show sex differences.

TABLE 4.2. SAMPLE OF MEDICATIONS THAT SHOW SEX DIFFERENCES

Medication	Reason Used
Acetaminophen	A painkiller
Alcohol	A sedative
Amitriptyline	An antidepressant
Chlordiazepoxide	An antianxiety medicine
Clozapine†	Treats severe schizophrenia
Diazepam†	Antianxiety medicine, tranquilizer
Flurazepam	A sleeping pill
Fluphenazine decanoate	Treats schizophrenia
Imipramine	An antidepressant
Lidocaine	An anesthetic
Lorazepam†	Antianxiety medicine, tranquilizer
Oxazepam	Antianxiety medicine, tranquilizer
Piroxicam‡	Fights inflammation, used in treating arthritis
Propranolol§	Treats high blood pressure
Temazepam	A sleeping pill
Thiothixene†	Treats psychotic disorders
Trazodone	An antidepressant

With the exception of trazodone, all these medications tend to be cleared faster from a man's body than from a woman's. Older men seem to have a slower clearance for trazodone than do women.

†This medication probably has sex differences.
‡This medication may have a sex difference in older persons.
§This medication may have a sex difference in younger persons.

What causes these variations? Some of the important factors in men and women that are known to affect medications include:

- Body size and weight
- Stomach emptying
- Secretion of stomach acids
- Lean body mass
- Body fat
- Total body water
- Blood flow to the brain
- Activity of enzymes in the liver
- Function of the kidneys

In some cases, the difference may be due to only one factor, such as weight. Many other times, however, sex differences are due to a combination of factors. This happens, for example, even when dosages are modified to reflect a woman's weight. Taken together, then, men and women may differ on average in many of the factors that affect medication absorption, distribution, metabolism, and elimination.

Sometimes sex differences exist but have no real effect. The medication may have a large margin of safety, which means there is a wide safety zone between the amount that is effective and the amount that is dangerous. Thus, even if a woman has higher blood levels of the drug than a man, she does not have much of an increase in risk.

LIFE CHANGES AND DRUG EFFICACY

Over the years, the way a woman responds to medication changes according to the stage of her life cycle. Many of these changes are coordinated by hormones. Female hormones, such as estrogen, change throughout a woman's monthly menstrual period and provide a woman with the ability to have a child. They also affect her response to medication. When female hormones are prescribed for a woman—for example, for birth control or hormone replacement after menopause—they also can play a role in at least some women.

During the years that a woman is sexually active, medication can affect this part of her life (see "Medications Affecting Sexual Function"). As a woman ages, her response to medication changes again.

The Menstrual Cycle

The menstrual cycle probably does not affect how most women respond to medication. However, a small group of women—maybe 5–10 percent—do show menstrual effects.

In some cases, the blood level of a medication drops a few days before a woman has her period. Sometimes the blood level is so low that the medication isn't effective anymore. Women who have these premenstrual drops in medication effectiveness may need to take higher doses of a medication before their periods, but this should be discussed first with the doctor. Once the period is over, they can go back to their regular doses. Other women find that their medications reach higher levels in the blood in the time before their periods. These women may have a higher risk of side effects.

If you find that your period seems to affect how you respond to medicine, talk with your doctors. They can study your blood levels and help decide whether changing doses would help increase the medication's effectiveness or reduce the risk of side effects.

Pregnancy

Pregnancy affects how a woman responds to medication, and it may affect the fetus. Because of fears of harming the fetus, few studies have been done on the effects of medications in pregnant women. For obvious reasons, medication should be carefully chosen in pregnancy. Because so little is known, it is best to avoid medicines at this time, even those available without a prescription.

When a woman is pregnant, her body must produce not only enough blood for her needs but also enough to circulate through the fetus. A pregnant woman's blood volume may increase by about 20–30 percent. As a result, she retains fluid and her total body water increases. Because this extra fluid tends to water down, or dilute, any medicine she takes, higher doses may be needed during pregnancy. In some medicines, though, the effective level in the blood may be very close to the hazardous level (a narrow therapeutic index). During pregnancy, this can be risky. Pregnant women who must take these kinds of medicines should have their blood levels checked often.

Medication can affect the fetus if it can cross the placenta, the organ where nutrients and oxygen are delivered to the fetus from the mother's blood.

The 9 months of a normal pregnancy can be divided into three trimesters of 3 months each. Medications taken in the first trimester have the greatest risk of causing birth defects. While medicines taken later in pregnancy are less likely to cause birth defects, they can cause other problems like low birth weight or delayed development.

Tell your doctor as soon as you know you are pregnant. The doctor can explain what medicines are safe to use during pregnancy. If you have a serious medical condition that requires medication, often you can be switched to one that is safer for the fetus. For example, warfarin, an anticoagulant used to prevent blood clots, can cause birth defects if used in pregnancy. Pregnant women who need to use an anticoagulant can choose heparin instead, which poses less risk to the unborn child. In some cases, it is believed that certain drugs (e.g., tricyclic antidepressants, but not lithium) are relatively safe during pregnancy. Even when such medications in pregnancy have not been formally tested, some women have taken the drug before they knew they were pregnant. Such information helps establish whether to take certain drugs in pregnancy. Work with your doctor to weigh the risks *and* benefits of medication use during pregnancy, for both mother and child.

Women who choose to breast-feed should be aware that medications can be excreted in breast milk and passed on to the baby. If you are breast-feeding, have any medication cleared by your physician (obstetrician or pediatrician) before taking it.

Menopause

The possible effects of menopause on various medications is largely unknown. What *is* known is that at menopause, a woman's blood levels of estrogen drop dramatically. This development can contribute to annoying symptoms such as hot flashes and can increase the risk of weak bones (osteoporosis) or heart disease. To replace the estrogen their bodies once made naturally, some women choose to take synthetic hormones. These hormones are sometimes similar to the ones in birth control pills, so their effects may resemble those of pills.

Birth Control and Medication

Certain birth control methods contain synthetic hormones similar to the ones a woman's body makes naturally, including:

- Birth control pills
- Hormone injections
- Hormone implants

Contraceptives like these can affect other medications or results on lab tests. If you use one of these methods, be sure to tell any doctor who prescribes medicine for you.

About 25 percent of U.S. women 15–45 years of age use birth control pills. The estrogen and progestin (a synthetic version of progesterone, a natural female hormone) in the pills can affect how the liver functions. When a woman who uses the pill takes other medications that are metabolized through the liver,

MEDICATIONS AFFECTING SEXUAL FUNCTION

Medication	Reason Used	Effect on Sexuality
Alprazolam	Treatment of anxiety	Changes in sex drive, sexual problems
Amiodarone	Corrects irregular heartbeat	Decreased sex drive
Atenolol	Lowers high blood pressure	Decreased sex drive
Amitriptyline	Antidepressant	Increased or decreased sex drive
Clofibrate	Lowers fat levels like cholesterol in the blood	Decreased sex drive
Clonidine	Lowers high blood pressure	Decreased sexual activity, decreased sex drive
Danazol	Treatment of endometriosis or fibrocystic breast disease	Vaginal dryness, increased or decreased sex drive
Diazepam	Treatment of anxiety	Changes in sex drive, sexual problems

Medication	Reason Used	Effect on Sexuality
Fenfluramine	Used in weight-loss programs	Increased or decreased sex drive
Fluoxetine	Antidepressant	Decreased sex drive, painful intercourse
Guanabenz	Lowers high blood pressure	Decreased sex drive
Methadone	Detox treatment for heroin abuse	Decreased sex drive
Methyldopa	Lowers high blood pressure	Decreased sex drive
Mexiletine	Corrects irregular heartbeat	Decreased sex drive
Nafarelin	Treatment of endometriosis	Vaginal dryness, decreased sex drive
Nifedipine	Relieves the chest pain of angina	Can cause sexual difficulties
Phentermine	Used in weight-loss programs	Changes in sex drive
Protriptyline	Antidepressant	Increased or decreased sex drive

Sources: S. M. Wolfe and R. E. Hope, Public Citizen Health Research Group. *Worst Pills Best Pills II* (Washington, DC: Public Citizen's Health Research Group, 1993) (for drug names); *Physicians' Desk Reference*, 48th ed. (Montvale, N.J.: Medical Economics Data Production Company, 1994) (for description of effect and confirmation of interaction)

she may have higher blood levels and more toxic side effects than a woman who uses other methods of birth control or no birth control at all. In this case, the pills exaggerate the differences that already exist because of the difference in sex. The effect may be greatest for pills with high amounts of progestin.

A birth control pill that contains only progestin (the minipill) is available. Hormone injections and implants also contain only progestin. Inform your doctor if you are taking birth control pills.

See Table 4.4 for more information.

Older Women

Medication is a particularly important issue for women over 65. In general, both metabolism and elimination of medications are slower in older people. The elderly tend to weigh less, too, so they may need less of a drug. Their livers and kidneys may not work as well, and they may have problems clearing medicines out of their systems. And even healthy older women are more sensitive to the effects of medicine.

The effects of age seem to be greater in men than in women, however, which means that older women may not need as low a dose after all. Generally, doctors should choose the right dose to use on the basis of each woman's needs, rather than use a standard dose for everyone.

Another problem is multiple medications. Older women tend to have more health problems than younger women, and they may be on a variety of drugs. For example, an older woman may suffer from diabetes, heart trouble, and arthritis. She could easily be taking a different medicine for each problem. These medications may have side effects, and they may interact with each other.

These interactions are more likely if a woman sees several different doctors, all of whom are prescribing medication for her. None of them may know what the others have prescribed. If you take a number of medicines, note all of them on a card that you keep with you. Better yet, make sure that a copy of your list is presented to any and all doctors at each visit. This precaution will help doctors to prescribe the right medicines for you.

It is also wise to talk periodically with your doctor about whether all of the drugs you are using are really needed. Some may even result in tolerance and addiction if they are used too long. If medication is stopped, sometimes annoying and debilitating symptoms will disappear on their own. Others, like insomnia, may be relieved by lifestyle changes such as getting more exercise and limiting beverages containing caffeine. Don't be afraid to question your doctor. You have a right to ask questions about the treatment you are receiving. If your physician is not responsive, find another one who is.

Taking medicines as prescribed is often a problem for the elderly who may have poor and declining sight. Plus, the more medicines she has to remember, the more likely she is to forget to take one or mix up her instructions. Making a list each night of all the medicines to be taken the next day and noting when to take them can help. Another alternative is to use a daily or weekly pill box dispenser. In some cases a family member can help to fill the pill box properly.

Sadly, some families actually encourage an old person to take more medications. Rather than spending time with a woman who complains about her aches and pains, her family and doctors may suggest that she take tranquilizers, sleeping pills, or antidepressants to make her feel better. Actually these only make her easier to handle. That's not a good reason to take medications, nor is it good medicine.

GETTING THE MOST FROM YOUR MEDICATIONS

When you buy an over-the-counter medication at a drugstore or a grocery, you frequently have the option of buying the less expensive store brand or the brand name. Often, you have the same choice with prescription medicines: you can buy the generic version or the brand name. It costs a lot to develop and advertise a new drug, so the price of a new, brand-name medication may be high. Initially only the company that developed the medicine is allowed to make it, so it can set the price as high as the market will bear.

After a medicine has been available for some time, other companies are allowed to produce their own versions. These generic versions must have the same basic effects as the brand-name variety but, by law, generic medicines are allowed to vary a little bit in the bioavailability of their active ingredients. The bioavailability may be a bit higher or lower. This small difference does not matter for many medications, and generics are often far less expensive than name-brand drugs. Some medications, however, such as some birth control pills and heart medications, require very specific blood levels of the medicine for safe use. If you must take these kinds of drugs, think carefully before you request a generic version. Also, certain psychoactive drugs may differ in bioavailability.

The active ingredient is only a small portion of each pill. The rest is made up of various fillers. Generic medicines are allowed to have different fillers than the brand-name product. If you are intolerant of any of the common medication fillers, such as lactose (milk sugar), or of certain dyes, or you need to watch your intake of salt, sugar, or alcohol, ask your doctor or pharmacist about the fillers used in the generic version.

Generics are a good choice, especially if cost is a concern. In many states and many health plans, a pharmacy will fill a prescription with a generic version unless the doctor specifically requests the brand name.

When selecting an over-the-counter drug or picking up a prescription medicine from the pharmacy, be sure that the medicine has not been tampered with (see "Signs of Medication Tampering"). If a box, container, or medicine shows signs of tampering, do not buy it. If you only discover the problem at home, do not use the medicine. Take it back immediately to the store or pharmacy and ask for a replacement.

SIGNS OF MEDICATION TAMPERING

Before buying or using any medication, whether an over-the-counter product or a prescription medication, check the following:

- Are the inner and outer wrappings tight and secure?
- Does the container appear to be too full or not full enough?
- Are the expiration date, lot number, and other information the same on the container and its outer wrapping or box?
- Is a liquid medicine the normal color and thickness?
- Do tablets look different than they usually do (unusual spots, dull and rough instead of shiny and smooth)?
- Do tablets all have the same imprint?
- Do capsules look cracked or dented?
- Does the medicine smell or taste different than usual?

SOURCE: Adapted from United States Pharmacopeial Convention, *United States Pharmacopeia,* DI vol. II, *Advice for the Patient: Drug Information in Lay Language* (Rockville, Md.: USPC, 1993).

Safe Medication Use

The most important thing you can do when taking medications is to take them as directed. Doing so increases the chance that the medication works as it's supposed to, and decreases the risk of side effects. Taking extra medicine because "it doesn't seem to be working" can be very risky. Stopping medication early because symptoms have cleared up can cause problems, too. For example, if you are being treated for an infection, it is very important that you take all the medication prescribed for you. If antibiotics (the common treatment for infections) are stopped early, the infection may come back. The bacteria causing the infection may then build up resistance, so that the same antibiotic doesn't work as well later, if you need it (see "What a Woman Needs to Know About Her Medicines").

Be prepared to tell a doctor about all other medicines you are taking, including those that can be bought without a prescription. As suggested earlier, you can jot this information down on a small card that you carry in your wallet. The card should also include any medical conditions you may have, along with any allergies to medicine.

Many medicines can interact with each other, or with food or alcohol. Be aware of any possible interactions with the medicine you've been prescribed. If medications that have the same type of effect are taken together, the effect can be greater than desired. For example, both alcohol and sleeping pills slow down the nervous system. If these products are taken together, the system can falter dangerously. Many deaths have resulted from this lethal combination.

On the other hand, products that have opposite effects reduce each other's effectiveness. For example, if a barbiturate is taken with a stimulant, such as a diet pill, these two types of medication may cancel each other out (see Tables 4.3–4.5). This type of up-down treatment is hard on the body too.

What a Woman Needs to Know About Her Medicines

To the extent possible, there are a number of things you should know about each medicine you are taking, including:

- The medicine's generic and brand names. This can be overwhelming.
- How it will help you and the expected results. How it makes you feel. How long it takes to begin working.
- How much to take at one time.
- How often to take the medicine.
- How long it will be necessary to take the medicine.
- When to take it. Before, during, after meals? At bedtime? At any other special times?
- How to take it. With water? With fruit juice? How much?
- What to do about a missed dose.
- Foods, drinks, or other medicines not to be taken while taking a medicine.
- Restrictions on activities while taking a medicine. May you drive or operate other motor vehicles?
- Side effects to be expected. What to do if they appear. How to minimize them. How soon should they go away? Insist that the physician give you side effects *in writing* (AMA sells these to doctors).

- When to seek help, if there are problems.
- How long to wait before reporting no change in symptoms.
- How to store the medicine. Should the unused portion be saved for future use?
- The expiration date.
- The cost of the medicine.
- How to have the prescription refilled, if necessary.

SOURCE: Adapted from United States Pharmacopeial Convention, *United States Pharmacopeia,* DI vol. II, *Advice for the Patient: Drug Information in Lay Language* (Rockville, Md.: USPC, 1993).

Reading a Prescription

It's only natural to want to know what you're putting in your body, so it may be important for you to be able to read prescriptions your doctors hand you.

Unfortunately, reading a prescription isn't quite as simple as reading a label. A prescription may look like it's written in a foreign language because it is. Prescriptions have their own set of abbreviations and codes, many of which are based on Latin. Being able to read a prescription can help you double-check that you're being given the instructions the doctor intended.

This list includes some of the terms that show up most often on prescriptions:

ac	Before meals (ante cibum)
ad	Right ear (auris dextra)
ad	Up to (ad)
ad lib	As desired (ad libitum)
as	Left ear (auris sinistra)
bid	Twice a day (bis in die)

c	With (cum)
et	And (et)
gtt(s)	Drop(s) (gutta)
h *or* **hr**	Hour (hora)
hs	At bedtime (hora somni)
M	Mix (misce)
nr	Do not repeat (non repetatur)
od	Right eye (oculus dexter)
os	Left eye (oculus sinister)
pc	After meals (post cibum)
po	By mouth (per os)
prn	As needed (pro re nata)
q	Each (quaque)
qd	Each day (quaque die)
qh *or* **q hr**	Each hour (quaque hora)
qid	Four times a day (quarter in die)
s	Without (sine)
ss	One-half (semis)
Sig	Mark, write (signa)
stat	At once (statim)
tid	Three times a day (ter in die)
ud *or* **ut dict**	As directed (ut dictum)

SAFE STORAGE OF MEDICATIONS

The bathroom cabinet may be a convenient place to store medicines, but the hot, steamy environment of a bathroom can make them break down into other products that can be useless or even dangerous. Store most medicines at room temperature in a dry, dark place. Don't store a medicine in the refrigerator unless the label says to do so.

All medications should be thrown away once you have taken the prescribed amount. Self-treating with old medications or with drugs prescribed for someone else is dangerous. Over-the-counter products like painkillers should be thrown out once their expiration date has passed.

Store medications away from children and pets. Today, many medications come in child-proof containers. If you find that the container is adult-proof as well, and there are no children in the house, your pharmacy can usually provide you with a regular container instead. It may be best to flush old or extra medicine down the toilet rather than leaving it in the trash for a child or pet to find.

TABLE 4.3. SAMPLE MEDICATION INTERACTIONS WITH FOOD

Medication	Reason Used	Foods That Interact	Effect of Interaction
Isoniazid	Treatment of tuberculosis	Cheese or fish	In some people causes sweating, chills, headache, faintness and palpitations, and red, itchy skin
Lithium	Treatment of manic depression	Sodium; coffee, tea	Lithium levels can be affected by rapid changes in amount of salt in diet; large amounts of tea or coffee can cause lithium to build up
Methoxsalen	Treatment of severe psoriasis (skin condition)	Limes, figs, parsley, parsnips, mustard, carrots, celery	May increase sensitivity of skin to light

Medication	Reason Used	Foods That Interact	Effect of Interaction
Monoamine-oxidase inhibitors (e.g., isocarboxazide, phenelzine)*	Treatment of depression	Foods high in tyramine (red wine, beer, some cheeses, fava beans, herring, and chocolate)	Can cause a serious rise in blood pressure
Potassium-sparing diuretics (for example, amiloride, spironolactone)	Increases the excretion of urine	Foods high in potassium (dried fruit and salt substitutes)	Potassium could rise to dangerous levels in the body
Tetracycline	Antibiotic	Milk products	Milk reduces absorption of tetracycline

Source: C. B. Clayman, *The American Medical Association Guide to Prescription and Over-the-Counter Drugs* (New York: Random House, 1988).

*Procarbazine, a medication used in cancer treatment, can have similar effects.

TABLE 4.4. SOME MEDICATION-MEDICATION INTERACTIONS

Medication (Reason Used)	Interacts with (Reason Used)	Type of Interaction
Amantadine (treatment of Parkinson's disease)	Anticholinergics (treatment of urinary incontinence and irritable bowel syndrome)	Increased effect of anticholinergics
Antacids (relieve stomach upset)	Digitalis (treatment of heart failure)	Reduced absorption of digitalis
	Iron (treatment of anemia, also found in multivitamins)	Reduced absorption of iron
	Isoniazid (treatment of tuberculosis)	Antacids containing aluminum can reduce absorption of isoniazid
	Quinine (treatment of malaria)	Antacids containing aluminum can reduce absorption of quinine
	Tetracycline (antibiotic)	Reduced absorption of tetracycline

Medication (Reason Used)	Interacts with (Reason Used)	Type of Interaction
Anticoagulants (prevent blood clotting)	Aspirin (painkiller)	Increased anticoagulant activity
	Barbiturates (sleeping pills)	Decreased anticoagulant activity
	Carbamazepine (prevents and controls seizures)	Decreased anticoagulant activity
	Chloramphenicol (antibiotic)	Increased anticoagulant activity
	Clofibrate (lowers fat levels like cholesterol in the blood)	Increased anticoagulant activity
	Griseofulvin (antifungal)	Decreased anticoagulant activity
	Thyroid hormones (adjust activity of thyroid gland)	Increased anticoagulant activity
Antidepressants, tricyclic (treatment of depression)	Barbiturates (sleeping pills)	May increase metabolism of antidepressants
	Guanethidine (lowers high blood pressure)	Decreased effectiveness of guanethidine
	Monoamine oxidase inhibitors (antidepressants)	Serious effects on nervous system, including seizures and death

TABLE 4.4. SOME MEDICATION-MEDICATION INTERACTIONS *(continued)*

Medication (Reason Used)	Interacts with (Reason Used)	Type of Interaction
Antihistamines (treatment of colds and allergies)	Anticholinergics (treatment of urinary incontinence and irritable bowel syndrome)	Increased anticholinergic effects of antihistamine (dry mouth, etc.)
	Monoamine oxidase inhibitors (antidepressants)	Dangerous rise in blood pressure
Birth control pills (prevention of pregnancy)	Barbiturates (sleeping pills)	Decreased effectiveness of birth control
	Phenytoin (prevents and controls seizures)	Decreased effectiveness of birth control
	Rifampin (antibacterial used in treatment of tuberculosis)	Decreased effectiveness of birth control
	Tricyclic antidepressants	Increased blood levels of the antidepressant may occur and dosage may need to be decreased.

Medication (Reason Used)	Interacts with (Reason Used)	Type of Interaction
Cephalosporins (antibiotics)	Aminoglycosides (antibiotics)	Possibly increased risk of kidney damage
	Probenecid (treatment of gout)	Increased level of cephalosporin in blood
Digoxin	Indomethacin	Rise in digoxin level (could be toxic)
Propranolol (treatment of high blood pressure, angina, and irregular heartbeat)	Cimetidine (treatment of ulcers)	Increased levels of propranolol in blood
	Indomethacin (relieves pain and inflammation)	Reduced effectiveness of propranolol
Pseudoephedrine (nasal decongestant)	Antihypertensives (reduce blood pressure)	Decreased effectiveness of antihypertensive
	Monoamine oxidase inhibitors (antidepressants)	Dangerous rise in blood pressure

Source: C. B. Clayman, *The American Medical Association Guide to Prescription and Over-the-Counter Drugs* (New York: Random House, 1988); J. E. Knoben and P. O. Anderson, *Handbook of Clinical Drug Data*, 5th ed. (Hamilton, Ill.: Drug Intelligence Publications, 1983).

TABLE 4.5 MEDICATION INTERACTIONS WITH ALCOHOL

Drug Name	Reason Used	Interaction with Alcohol
Aspirin	Headaches and other body pain, blood thinner	Increased risk of bleeding in the stomach or intestines
Disulfiram	In alcohol treatment programs to develop aversion to alcohol	Dilation (expansion) of veins, low blood pressure, headache, breathing problems, nausea, vomiting, chest pain, weakness, and confusion
Methotrexate	Cancer treatment, rheumatoid arthritis, psoriasis	Increases methotrexate's risk of liver damage
Metronidazole	Fungal infections, such as vaginal infections	Reactions similar to those with disulfiram
Nitroglycerin	To treat pain of angina	Both drugs dilate (expand) the veins, so low blood pressure may occur
Phenytoin	To prevent seizures	Phenytoin more rapidly metabolized with long-term use of large amounts of alcohol

Source: Condensed from J. E. Knoben and P. O. Anderson, *Handbook of Clinical Drug Data,* 5th ed. (Hamilton, Ill.: Drug Intelligence Publications, 1983).

EDITORS AND CONTRIBUTORS

MEDICAL CO-EDITORS

ROSELYN PAYNE EPPS, M.D., M.P.H., M.A., F.A.A.P., is an expert at the National Institutes of Health, Bethesda, Maryland, and a Professor at Howard University College of Medicine, Washington, D.C. She is recognized nationally and internationally in areas of health policy and research, health promotion and disease prevention, and medical education and health service delivery. As a pioneer and leader in numerous professional and community organizations, she served, in 1991, as the first African-American president of AMWA and the founding president of the AMWA foundation.

SUSAN COBB STEWART, M.D., F.A.C.P., is an internist and gastroenterologist, and is presently Associate Medical Director at J. P. Morgan in New York, where she delivers general medical care, specialty consultations, and preventive services. She is Clinical Assistant Professor of Medicine at SUNY, Brooklyn. Since serving as president of AMWA in 1990, Dr. Stewart has continued to help AMWA shape and focus its mission in the area of women's health.

CONTRIBUTORS

Claudia R. Baquet, M.D., M.P.H., serves as Visiting Scholar in Health Policy and Assistant Dean for Health Affairs at the University of Maryland School of Medicine in Baltimore, Maryland. She developed and implemented the first national cancer prevention and control intervention research program that focuses solely on African-American and Native American populations.

Kathleen M. Foley, M.D., is attending Neurologist at both Memorial Sloan-Kettering Cancer Center and New York Hospital. She is a Professor of Neurology and

Neuroscience and of Clinical Pharmacology at Cornell University Medical College. Further, she serves as a Consultant at Rockefeller University Hospital and Calvary Hospital.

Jean A. Hamilton, M.D., is a Professor of Psychology, Social and Health Sciences, and Women's Studies at Duke University and an Associate Professor in Psychiatry and Consultant to the general internal medicine section's "Women's Health Program" at Duke University Medical Center, Durham, North Carolina. She cofounded and served as Director of the Institute for Research on Women's Health.

Janet Rose Osuch, M.D., F.A.C.S., is an Associate Professor of Surgery and Medical Director of the Comprehensive Breast Health Clinic at Michigan State University. She is Chair of the Breast Cancer Subcommittee of AMWA and is American Cancer Society Breast Cancer Subcommittee Chair and National Spokesperson on breast cancer.

Kimberly A. Yonkers, M.D., trained in psychiatry and psychopharmacology, currently works in the Departments of Psychiatry and Obstetrics and Gynecology at the University of Texas Southwestern Medical Center, Dallas. Her work is focused on elucidating hormonal influences on affective disorders in women.

INDEX